"*The Brain Trust Program* provides everything you need to know to ensure optimal brain functioning for a lifetime!"

—Christiane Northrup, M.D., author of *Women's Bodies, Women's Wisdom*;
The Wisdom of Menopause; and *Mother-Daughter Wisdom*

"It isn't difficult to find people who are suffering from a wide range of debilitating neurological conditions such as migraine headaches, Alzheimer's disease, brain cancer, and worse these days. But leave it to a brain surgeon to figure out many of these can actually be treated and even reversed metabolically through some rather simple changes in the diet. Dr. Larry McCleary has figured out that controlling the amount of insulin production by consuming a healthy low-carb diet is indeed the most "brain-friendly" way you could possibly eat. The Brain Trust Program he has developed from his many years of experience challenges people to think about the long-term impact of the high-carb foods they are eating not just on their waistline, but also on that gray matter between their ears! This book is guaranteed to shake up the status quo and quite literally turn traditional brain treatment on its head!"

—Jimmy Moore, author of *Livin' La Vida Low-Carb*

"One of the best books I've seen on the care and feeding of your brain! Dr. McCleary knows what he's talking about and, even better, has a gift for communicating this important information!"

—Jonny Bowden, Ph.D., CNS Board Certified Nutritionist,
author of *The 150 Healthiest Foods on Earth* and
The Most Effective Natural Cures on Earth

The Brain Trust Program

A scientifically based

three-part plan to improve

memory, elevate mood,

enhance attention, alleviate

migraine and menopausal

symptoms, and boost

mental energy

Larry McCleary, M.D.

A Perigee Book

A PERIGEE BOOK
Published by the Penguin Group
Penguin Group (USA) Inc.
375 Hudson Street, New York, New York 10014, USA
Penguin Group (Canada), 90 Eglinton Avenue East, Suite 700, Toronto, Ontario M4P 2Y3, Canada
(a division of Pearson Penguin Canada Inc.)
Penguin Books Ltd., 80 Strand, London WC2R 0RL, England
Penguin Group Ireland, 25 St. Stephen's Green, Dublin 2, Ireland (a division of Penguin Books Ltd.)
Penguin Group (Australia), 250 Camberwell Road, Camberwell, Victoria 3124, Australia
(a division of Pearson Australia Group Pty. Ltd.)
Penguin Books India Pvt. Ltd., 11 Community Centre, Panchsheel Park, New Delhi—110 017, India
Penguin Group (NZ), 67 Apollo Drive, Rosedale, North Shore 0745, Auckland, New Zealand
(a division of Pearson New Zealand Ltd.)
Penguin Books (South Africa) (Pty.) Ltd., 24 Sturdee Avenue, Rosebank, Johannesburg 2196, South Africa

Penguin Books Ltd., Registered Offices: 80 Strand, London WC2R 0RL, England

While the author has made every effort to provide accurate telephone numbers and Internet addresses at the time of publication, neither the publisher nor the author assumes any responsibility for errors, or for changes that occur after publication. Further, the publisher does not have any control over and does not assume any responsibility for author or third-party websites or their content.

First edition: September 2007

Library of Congress Cataloging-in-Publication Data

McCleary, Larry.
   The brain trust program : a scientifically based three-part plan to improve memory, elevate mood, enhance attention, alleviate migraine and menopausal symptoms, and boost mental energy / Larry McCleary.— 1st ed.
       p.   cm.
   "A Perigee book."
   Includes bibliographical references.
   ISBN 978-0-399-53358-7
   1. Brain—Popular works.   2. Brain—care and hygiene—Popular works.   I. Title.
   QP376.M12   2007
   612.8'2—dc22

                                                                              2007017536

PRINTED IN THE UNITED STATES OF AMERICA

10   9   8   7   6   5   4   3   2   1

PUBLISHER'S NOTE: Neither the publisher nor the author is engaged in rendering professional advice or services to the individual reader. The ideas, procedures, and suggestions contained in this book are not intended as a substitute for consulting with your physician. All matters regarding your health require medical supervision. Neither the author nor the publisher shall be liable or responsible for any loss or damage allegedly arising from any information or suggestion in this book. The names and identifying characteristics of patients have been changed to protect their privacy.

Most Perigee books are available at special quantity discounts for bulk purchases for sales promotions, premiums, fund-raising, or educational use. Special books, or book excerpts, can also be created to fit specific needs. For details, write: Special Markets, Penguin Group (USA) Inc., 375 Hudson Street, New York, New York 10014.

To Christine

ACKNOWLEDGMENTS

First and foremost I would like to thank my patients and their parents whose quiet courage in consenting to proceed with brain surgery, often knowing me only for minutes, is both touching and overwhelming. What they have taught me has made me a better physician.

I would also like to acknowledge multiple invaluable conversations with Dr. Mary Dan Eades, a dear friend and colleague.

Last, but certainly not least, I would like to thank John Duff, from Perigee Books, for his thoughtful guidance and perspective, keen sense of humor, and continued encouragement so necessary for the development and formulation of this manuscript.

CONTENTS

INTRODUCTION

During a typical working day as a brain surgeon, Dr. Larry McCleary spent hours probing and peering into the brains of his patients. He might have started by inserting a shunt into the ventricles positioned deep within the brain of a young patient to prevent fluid buildup and the resulting hydrocephalus. This may have been followed with a complicated operation to remove a precariously positioned tumor located deep within the cranium of another patient and then a quick trip to the emergency room to evaluate a youngster with head trauma. He might have finished the day with yet another surgery, operating up through the base of the skull to repair a malformed blood vessel. Or his day might have involved one of the 12- to 14-hour reparative surgeries that he so deftly performed. These many operations were always augmented by hours of postoperative follow-up, visting patients in the hospital and office and consulting with other physicians.

In fact, Dr. McCleary's life was like that of any hardworking pediatric neurosurgeon—with one major difference. Dr. McCleary not only probed the brain with his surgical instruments but probed the brain with his intellect. He devoted his time not just to making a diagnosis but also to studying what makes the brain really tick. Although he understood that removing a tumor or a blood-vessel malformation from the brain would solve a host of problems, he was driven to ensure that he gave the brains under his care the best chance of healing, growing, and developing normally. So, not only did he spend the time any neurosurgeon would on the study of his craft but he spent an enormous amount of time studying the metabolism of and the influence of nutrition and supplementation on the brain. We've known and worked with

Dr. McCleary for many years. Every time we see him, he shares with us the most recent scientific papers on nutrition and the brain. More important, he teaches us how this research applies to our own medical practice. We've been after him for years to share his lifetime of study, research, and clinical experience with a wider audience by putting it into a book. He's finally complied—and what a book it is.

In our specialty of nutritional medicine, we read dozens of books on all forms of diets and nutritional and nutraceutical supplementation. Included in these volumes are texts about improving the brain (or preventing or forestalling its decline with age). Most of these books present warmed-over recommendations to follow low-fat diets (often a disaster for an ailing or struggling brain), to take a few well-known vitamins, maybe (in the more enlightened books) to add some fish oil, and usually to do aerobic exercise. At best, these books show in general terms how to keep what you've got from deteriorating. At worst, they present checklists of diseases that arise when brains go bad, allowing readers to self-diagnose which sort of brain disorders afflict them but offering no clear recommendations for how to fix such problems. No book written by a neuroscientist, until this one, really deals with how to *improve* cognitive performance.

As both health-care providers and consumers, we want and need to understand the underlying problems. It is easy, for example, to compile an extensive list of symptoms of a heart attack: shortness of breath, profuse sweating, crushing chest pain, mottled skin, and so on. But what good does it do to simply be able to see a heart attack in progress, tick off all the signs, and say, "Yep, that's a heart attack all right." What we need to know is what's going on with the heart that causes all these signs and, more important, what we can do about it. It is the same with the brain. And what far too many books (and doctors) do is offer up lists of ever more sensitive diagnostic indicators of memory loss or Alzheimer's disease. Then, when these signs are present, they can tick them all off and say, "Yep, that's Alzheimer's."

No one wants to hear "Yep, that's Alzheimer's" when it's their own diagnosis or that of a loved one. Dr. McCleary's book is cut from a different bolt of cloth; it describes how to take proactive steps to avoid ever hearing those words. He shows how to take these steps by altering something that we all can control: the metabolic status of our own brain cells. Improved brain cell metabolism—the chemical changes by which energy is provided for vital processes within brain cells—means improved brain health. Improved brain health not only can improve brain function but can substantially reduce the risk of developing memory impairment and a host of other brain problems, including Alzheimer's disease. The Three-Step Brain Trust Program he offers here details his metabolic approach to brain health based on extensive experience accumulated while caring for thousands of very sick brains.

Our brain cells are postmitotic, which is science-speak meaning that these cells don't reproduce like most other cells in the body. The ones we are born with are the ones we will die with . . . or without, should we end up losing a bunch of them. Maintaining the same cells for a lifetime requires a much different protective strategy than that required for those cells that are constantly being sloughed off and replaced. Because they are around for only a few days, rapidly reproducing cells don't get the chance to accumulate much damage over time. Brain cells, however, don't work that way. Most of the neurons in your brain are as old as you are and have collected all the little dents and dings associated with the aging process. Think of your skin. It doesn't look the same as it did when you were in your teens and neither do your brain cells.

Aging brain cells lose some of their quickness and flexibility and, more important, some of their ability to continuously generate the high levels of energy they require to do all that they do. How much energy do they require? A lot. The entire brain constitutes about 2 percent of the weight of the body yet consumes 20 percent of the energy, which means that it is ten times more metabolically active than the rest of the body. One of the ways to provide fuel for the brain is to consume sugar—it provides a quick boost in short-term energy but at a long-term cost. People whose diet contains a large amount of sugar or foods that are rapidly turned into sugar frequently have blood sugar problems and also much, much higher rates of memory loss and other degenerative brain disorders, including Alzheimer's; the connection is quite clear. In *The Brain Trust Program*, Dr. McCleary tells how to avoid that Faustian bargain by using a combination of specific dietary and supplement recommendations to improve the brain's ability to generate the high energy levels it needs to function properly while maintaining proper glucose and insulin levels and thereby preventing the long-term damage that can accrue when these levels are chronically elevated.

Other evolving research links normal insulin metabolism and neurogenesis (the formation of new brain or nerve cells). Recent scientific findings have made it clear, contrary to years of opposite belief, that we in fact do have the ability to produce new nerve cells throughout our lives. It is also clear that these new nerve cells interact with others and become integrated into the fully functioning brain. And it's also known that as we age this process of neurogenesis slows down. Although these new findings have not yet been fully explored by neuroscientists, it is clear that the new brain cells are involved in memory, learning, emotion, and mood—the very skills and states that Alzheimer's disease affects. In fact, the first place that Alzheimer's strikes is the hippocampus, the gatekeeper for memory. What is now also understood is that this same area of the brain is strongly influenced by cortisol, the stress hormone. Chronically elevated levels of cortisol cause the death of brain cells that affect both memory and mood, a finding that has led researchers toward an entirely new way of thinking about mood disorders and their treatment. If we can stimulate the nerve growth factors necessary to build new brain cells while taking preventative steps to remove (or at least block the effects of) substances, such as cortisol, that are known to destroy brain cells, we can make huge strides in preventing memory loss and, at the same time, rev up the brain to work much better. The great news is that these are processes under metabolic control and hence something we can influence with the lifestyle choices we make. It is truly exciting that, with Dr. McCleary's groundbreaking Brain Trust Program, we now have the nutritional, supplemental, and cognitive tools necessary to encourage the growth of new nerve cells. None of this information has appeared in any brain book on the market and, in fact, even most physicians are not aware of it. Until now.

But it doesn't end there. Thanks to Dr. McCleary's wide-ranging research, this book proffers a new theory of and offers solutions for conditions most people would not at first blush consider brain problems: menopause and its symptoms. At present, most women approach their middle years with trepidation. In the recent past, women could minimize the symptoms of menopause—hot flashes, mood swings, anxiety, and brain fog—with the use of hormone-replacement therapy (HRT). Unfortunately, the newest research has shown that HRT is not benign. Women heading into menopause are now confronted with the difficult choice of simply enduring menopausal misery or undertaking a therapy now known to substantially increase risk for disease in the future. This book provides a third choice.

It turns out that the hot flashes, memory lapses, and other symptoms of menopause are brain driven. They are manifestations of energy disturbances in the brain that can be smoothed out with proper nutrition. *The Brain Trust Program* describes a groundbreaking new dietary solution to the discomfort that all too often accompanies what many women refer to as the curse of menopause.

Another curse that strikes people of all ages and both sexes is migraine headaches. Anyone who has not experienced the blinding pain and visual disruption of these headaches cannot imagine the discomfort and disability they cause. Migraines are also typically driven by disrupted brain metabolism—in this case, the imbalance of a couple of elements that regulate the firing of the clusters of brain cells involved. Here, too, Dr. McCleary provides relief not with medications but through nutrition. By consuming the proper balance of nutrients and brain supplements, migraine headaches can be conquered.

Those who read this book can be assured that they are receiving the most up-to-date, authoritative information available. This information is the synthesis of the knowledge contained in thousands of pages of medical and scientific literature, distilled by a first-rate neuroscientific mind and refined by years of clinical practice. Dr. McCleary has clearly written the most important brain improvement book to come along in many years. Read it and follow his recommendations. You will be rewarded with clearer, crisper cognition and be able to rest easy knowing that as long as you care for your brain, your brain will care for you.

—Michael R. Eades, MD, and Mary Dan Eades, MD

A Metabolic Approach to Brain Health

A Full Spectrum of Gray

Maude W's Brain Fog

Maude felt as if she were losing her edge. As president and CEO of an advertising agency, she was accustomed to the headaches that are an expected part of running a business and the necessity of being able to wear several hats at the same time. She'd always prided herself on her ability to multitask. The ease with which she could simultaneously juggle six different issues was almost legendary within the company. Lately, however, she found it more difficult to concentrate. Sometimes she couldn't find the exact word she wanted; she found herself jotting down dozens of notes to keep from forgetting something—and it wasn't always working. While none of these memory lapses was severe individually, together she felt they were compromising her ability to perform at the high level to which she and her clients were accustomed.

Lately she'd been under more stress than usual. There had been some unexpected financial twists this year and some troubling health issues with her mother, but nothing that would have thrown her in the past. At 57, she was worried that if she couldn't shake this brain fog, it might spell the end of her career, and she wasn't ready to get out of the business world quite yet. She wanted to know what she could do.

Because she and I had known each other for a number of years and because she knew that in addition to practicing neurosurgery I had an interest in the field of nutrition and brain health, she called me to see if I had any thoughts about her situation. I agreed with her assessment that stress was indeed a part of the problem, but both sleep deprivation (she was trying to get by on about 4.5 hours of sleep a night) and inadequate nutritional support compromised her ability to withstand the stress. I instructed her to begin immediately to aim for at least 7 hours of sleep each night, to delegate some responsibility to key employees at work, to restructure her day to permit some time for brain R&R, and to take a step back to look at and set priorities in different aspects of her life. In addition to these lifestyle changes, I recommended an antistress cocktail of nutrients designed to help her sleep more soundly; nourish her brain; help her handle the stress; focus more effectively; and maintain a stable, positive mood. Within weeks, she said that the fogginess was gone; she felt back in charge, her old self again.

It's important to understand that difficulty maintaining focus, multitasking meltdown, and memory decline don't merely exist in a black-and-white, you-have-it-or-you-don't fashion but as a full spectrum that ranges from the occasional senior moment to a total cognitive wipeout similar to that suffered by former President Ronald Reagan. The entire nation bore witness to his struggle and to Nancy Reagan's quiet strength in dealing with it. Today's active boomers have already begun to face similar scenarios with their own parents. In a very few years, without intervention, their own children will have to do likewise. The struggle to rehabilitate the injured or sick brain is an issue that I've dealt with for many years with patients, with colleagues, and now with friends.

During my years of clinical practice as a pediatric neurosurgeon, I primarily dealt with the extreme insults inflicted on young brains by accidents and disease: brains ravaged by the blunt trauma of car wrecks, falls, or abuse; brains injured by lack of oxygen from drowning, stroke, electrocution, or suffocation; brains damaged by tumors and the chemotherapy or irradiation used to combat them. Initially, most of them needed my surgical skills. Thereafter, almost without exception, they also required intense rehabilitation involving not only the standard occupational and physical therapies necessary for learning to walk and talk again but, as I came to understand, vital nutritional therapy to pave the way for success. Over years of medical practice, I learned that it was possible to vastly improve my patients' outcomes through the early and aggressive use of more than just the standard sugar water intravenous (IV) infusions given in the days before and after surgery and during recovery. I began including other nutrients critical to brain health—medium-chain triglycerides, amino acid mixtures, vitamins, minerals, and antioxidants—in my patients' IV formulas and then prescribing these nutrients and others to be taken in food and supplement form during the patients' ongoing recovery. And I noticed amazing results.

It was in this type of critical care setting where I first began to speculate that if proper care and feeding of the seriously injured brain and nervous system could make such a dramatic difference, what could it do for less serious insults? As time marched on for me and my fellow boomers, and I retired from my surgical practice, I shifted my focus to research, combing the medical and scientific literature to ferret out any known nutritional substance that would benefit the brain and nerves. My search added many more nutrients to my brain wellness pharmacopoeia: some of them exotic—such as *Huperzia serrata*, the active ingredient in a Chinese moss long used as a nerve tonic by Asian practitioners—others more pedestrian, but all of them shown in scientific studies to offer support for the brain and nerves and all of them available without a prescription. I became convinced that my program of brain health and nutrition could help combat the lesser insults that gradually accumulate simply as a consequence of living and many other situations as well.

Anita's Story

Anita N. had been stuck for hours in the traffic backed up on a snowy interstate highway and was finally making her way home when her car hit an icy patch and rolled over, pinning her in the driver's seat. She awoke on a ventilator in the intensive care unit (ICU) after undergoing emergency surgery to stabilize the three broken bones in her neck and to relieve the pressure on the severely damaged nerves supplying her right hand. After several weeks in the hospital and extensive therapy, she was able to walk with a walker; but she continued to experience severe weakness, numbness, and lack of coordination in her right arm. About 6 months later she was able to walk normally but could not hold a pen or feed herself with her right hand. More disturbing, she experienced a near-constant, unpleasant sensation that bugs were crawling all over her hand. Although I was her neighbor and not her doctor, but because she was frustrated that her recovery seemed to have hit a plateau, Anita contacted me to see if there was anything more that she could do.

As we spoke, I explained that there is currently no cure for a severed nerve or a way to resurrect brain cells once they have died. When sick or injured, nerve and brain cells react in similar ways and require similar types of nutritional support: first and foremost, they must be able to generate energy to support all the metabolic processes necessary for repair, recovery, and regeneration; they need to quell the inflammation that arises from exposure to a toxin, infection, or mechanical injury; and they have to stabilize and reorganize patterns of disordered and uncontrolled firing (which can better be thought of as electrical short-circuiting) that occur after such insults. I reassured her that there are nutrients that address each of these needs and that I would design a combination of them that I felt would help speed along her recovery. She began a regimen that included high levels of B vitamins to help the sick nerve cells generate the necessary energy for healing; various antioxidants and other natural anti-inflammatory agents to quiet the inflammation; and several botanical (plant-derived) compounds to improve the cells' ability to handle calcium, the proper channeling of which is critical for nerve impulse transmission.

Over a period of weeks, she gradually lost the creepy crawly feeling in her hand and noticed an increase in her sense of touch, something that had been missing since the accident. Soon after that, she began to recover intentional movement in her fingers and little by little regained control over what she did with her right hand. When I saw her about a year later, she was playing golf, typing, and doing all the things she had been able to do before her accident.

The Case of George B.

Jonathan B., the CEO of a biotech firm, had been at work when his wife, Betsy, called to tell him that his father, George, had gone for a walk in the neighborhood about 2 hours ago and had not returned. She had sent their teenage son, Jonah, to drive up and down the streets of their neighborhood searching for him. Jonah finally found his grandfather, about four blocks away, sitting on a bus bench at a busy intersection. When Jonah pulled up in the car, George seemed to recognize his face, but couldn't recall his name. Jonah was able to coax his grandfather into the car and drive him home, where he admitted to Betsy that he had forgotten where he was and couldn't remember the way back to the house. This marked the second time in as many weeks that George had become lost on his daily walk through a neighborhood in which he had lived for more than 20 years.

Just 2 years earlier, George had celebrated his 50th wedding anniversary with his college sweetheart when she unexpectedly passed away. In the wake of this sudden and staggering loss, George and his family acknowledged that he had become depressed. They sought medical attention for the depression; but, despite grief counseling and medication, he began to show signs of mental slippage. At first, it was just the typical things: misplaced keys and difficulty finding the car in a parking lot or recalling words or names. He and his family attributed these mild memory lapses—the kind many of us suffer now and again—to his depression or the effects of his antidepressant medications, but the symptoms progressed.

Before long, he found himself needing to read paragraphs in the newspaper over and over again, having trouble remembering what had just happened in a movie on TV, and being unable to recall his grandson's name. He had lost interest in reading, in watching TV or movies, and in visiting with his friends a few mornings a week at the local coffee shop. On the heels of these changes came the first episode of wandering lost in his own neighborhood, prompting Jonathan and Betsy to suggest that he move in with them.

After this most recent episode, Jonathan took his dad to the hospital, where his doctor performed a complete battery of lab tests and brain scans to rule out the possibility of stroke or other cause for George's disorientation and memory loss. The diagnosis was that George was suffering from early Alzheimer's disease, complicated by multiple small strokes over time and mild high blood pressure. In addition to treating George's blood pressure, his doctor felt that he would benefit from a structured environment and suggested providing him with a written schedule to help him cope with the mental changes. The family posted a daily agenda on the refrigerator along with reminders to turn off the burner on the stovetop. George began carrying a small spiral notebook and pen in his pocket to jot down phone calls he answered during the day and to record when he took his medication. These measures helped a bit, but his family wondered what more they might do.

Jonathan and I have had a passing business acquaintance over the years; and knowing about my expertise in brain health, he called me to see what my thoughts were on his father's situation. I explained that since I was far away it was critical to keep his own doctor there abreast of their concerns and to have George seen regularly; but that, yes, there were indeed a number of other treatments that I felt would be of help. I laid out a program of dietary change and nutritional supplementation designed to sharpen George's mental focus, improve his ability to remember, lift the fogginess, and restore his sense of well-being. The scientist in Jonathan wanted research citations, which I happily gave to him (and which are included in the bibliography on page 225).

After he had done his homework, Jonathan called me again to tell me how pleasantly surprised he had been to discover the extent of published information about the nutrients I had recommended; he was doubly pleased that they all appeared to be not only safe but good for the body in general. His father's doctor had reviewed the proposed regimen and given his okay, saying that he could see no harm in trying, though he didn't hold out much hope that the nutrients would offer much help. Jonathan told him that hope was about all he had going right now and he was surprised that no one on his father's medical team had suggested any of them.

Cautiously optimistic, he started his dad on my prescribed nutrient regimen (the details of which you'll find in later chapters). About 10 weeks later, Jonathan left me an urgent message to call him. I feared something had happened to his dad, yet when I called back, I was delighted to learn that not only was George tolerating the program but, in Jonathan's words, he was "acting like a new man." He had become much more socially interactive, his old sense of humor had returned, he could enjoy watching a movie with the family, and he was even able to have meaningful conversations with his grandson (whose name he could now usually recall) about what the boy was learning at school. Most important, he felt good about himself again. By nourishing his brain properly, George had been able to take back control of his life in meaningful ways. Now a year and a half later, he continues to do well; and through a thoughtful combination of diet and nutrient supplementation, George has even been safely weaned off his blood pressure medication.

While many responses aren't this dramatic, in my experience, the case of George B. is not unusual; it is the expected result of the proper care and feeding of the brain. It serves to illustrate that we have the understanding and ability to forestall, or to a large degree prevent, the looming tsunami of memory deficit that, if not addressed, will soon begin to engulf the aging boomers and, because of their vast numbers, wreck economic havoc on the strained national budget and swamp an already overburdened health-care system. Studies show that simply forestalling the onset of Alzheimer's disease by a single year could save an estimated $20 billion in health-care and associated costs. It can be done, and this book will show you exactly how.

The temples of all of America's baby boomers are now graying, with the youngest members of this group of nearly 78 million people having passed the big 4-0. Those on the leading edge of the boom blew out 60 candles in the year 2006. Although this generation has displayed great devotion to maintaining its youthful appearance, beneath the tinted roots and Botox-ed brows lay 78 million aging brains that most boomers are currently doing nothing to preserve and potentially much to injure.

Current statistical information tells us that with age comes an increased likelihood of mental decline. As David Brooks correctly pointed out in an October 2, 2005, *New York Times* editorial piece, a staggering 40 percent of us will suffer some form of dementia—among boomers, this figure will translate into nearly 32 million people unable to find their keys and futilely searching their memory banks for the right word or someone's name. About 10 percent of the over-65 population will have a slightly greater degree of mental decline, called mild cognitive impairment (MCI). This group will include nearly 8 million boomers, who will experience greater and more persistent memory deficits similar to those seen in mild Alzheimer's disease. After the boomers begin to hit age 65, some of them (statistically about 15 percent each year of those with MCI) will go on to develop full-blown Alzheimer's disease, suffering severe impairment in memory and thinking that will substantially interfere with their ability to live independently. Most of these people will require medication and assisted living care, which will place an enormous emotional and financial burden on the country because of this group's sheer numbers.

Reason to Hope

Age takes its toll on both man and machine; that's not news. Joints creak, arteries narrow, eyesight dims, skin wrinkles, waistlines expand, and chests sag. The longer we live, the longer time and gravity have to exert their effects. And more of us are living substantially longer. Children born in 1900 could expect to live 47.9 years if male and 50.7 years if female. A century later, advances in medical science project figures of 74.1 years for men and 79.5 for women. In the course of our lives, we accumulate a portfolio of dents and dings throughout the body: We may drink too much, to the detriment of our livers; we may eat poorly, to the detriment of our hearts and waistlines; and we may smoke, to the detriment of just about everything. We can modify these risk factors pretty easily if we choose to. Most of us grudgingly do so as the clock ticks by and the ravages of time become apparent on lab tests, on the scale, and in the mirror. Although doing what is good for the body in nutrition and lifestyle will generally be good for the brain as well, there are additional brain-specific measures that we could and should take, if we're to preserve this most critical organ in its best possible shape to the end of what we hope are very long, productive lives.

The brain is like every other organ in the body, only more so. It's more delicate, more metabolically active, more easily damaged, requires more energy, and is more in need of serious nutritional and lifestyle support if it's to stay fit longer. Unfortunately, it's an area of our health we can easily ignore, because the consequences of brain aging aren't something we can readily see by looking in the mirror or stepping on the scale; there's no neat little lab test that can quickly pinpoint risk.

Prior scientific dogma taught us that as we age, brain and nerve cells die. We are now beginning to understand that long before cell death occurs, subtle changes rewire the connections between brain cells, eventually robbing them of their ability to communicate effectively with one another. In other words, loss of our mental edge sneaks up on us, but we've laid the groundwork for it throughout life. The good news is that it's not too late; *until the brain cells actually perish, we can still intervene!* Learning how to properly feed and care for your brain can slow or even reverse the mental decline that age brings to us all—some of us more severely than others. It can even sharpen the focus of younger brains, as I have witnessed many times throughout my career.

Christopher's Story

Christopher was a 19-year-old college freshman, facing midterm exams for the first time. Overwhelmed by the sheer volume of information he'd been expected to digest, he was coming to grips with the reality that his study skills were not as efficient or productive as they could be. Sleep deprived and stressed out, he was subsisting on junk food and caffeine, which only served to make him jittery and unable to sleep when he had the chance to catch some much-needed rack time. Since I had known his mom for many years, she recommended that Chris give me a call to see what he could do. When he contacted me, he told me he needed something that worked and worked fast.

Chris needed help learning how to relax to relieve the stress that was certainly contributing to his woes, and I instructed him in some techniques to do that. Reluctantly, he agreed to give up junk food in favor of the fish, meat, dairy, fruits, and veggies in the cafeteria line; he was that desperate. But at this point, his brain needed more than just nutritious food to be able to focus his concentration for prolonged periods of study. Certainly, that's something that caffeine does for many people. Coffee has even been linked to a decreased risk for developing Alzheimer's disease, but it wasn't a suitable choice for Chris; he couldn't tolerate the jittery side effects. Instead, I designed a regimen that included increased doses of certain B vitamins, a network of antioxidants, such as α-lipoic acid and coenzyme Q10 (CoQ_{10}), a pretty hefty dose of magnesium, and some dimethylaminoethanol (DMAE) and huperzine A. These last ingredients have been shown in clinical trials to increase prolonged focus when taken in sufficient amounts.

A few weeks later, he was able to face his midterms and even did pretty well on them. The longer he stayed on the program, the more effectively he was able to focus on his studies and refine his study techniques; by the end of the term, he even aced several of his exams. His dramatic turnaround created converts to the brain wellness support plan among his friends. During the last contact I had with Chris, I learned he was applying to grad school.

Diet and lifestyle choices we make early in life clearly have an effect on the development of disease later in life. The connections are especially evident in the realms of obesity, heart disease, high blood pressure, and diabetes. We now understand that obese kids grow up to become obese adults; we've witnessed college jocks grow into businessmen with bloated bellies and triple bypasses. But what may be less obvious is the effect of how we eat and what we do on our ability to perceive, think, focus, remember, and react. It is very clear today that the life we are living can put us at greater risk to lose these abilities sooner than we ought. We expend great energy and money preserving our bodies but precious little to support the very thing that most sets us apart as human. Consider the words of René Descartes: I think, therefore, I am. If we are unable to think, then what are we?

Preserving (even improving) your senses, your mental sharpness, and your memory is possible; in fact, it's pretty painless. In the subsequent chapters, I'll show you how to assess your current degree of risk for age-associated memory loss, mild cognitive impairment, or Alzheimer's disease. You'll also discover what to do and why.

2

Why the Brain Is Vulnerable: The Goldilocks Principles

I've spent the better part of my life studying the human brain, investigating how it's made, teasing it apart, putting it back together, appreciating all that it does, and understanding why it's perhaps the most vulnerable—and valuable—of all our organs. Sometimes in my job as a brain surgeon that meant physically trying to piece together damaged parts to restore the best possible function. An intimate working knowledge of the structure and function of the brain is, obviously, of great importance to a brain surgeon trying to nurture an injured or sick brain back to good health. But I contend that, because knowledge is power, it behooves *all* of us who desire to improve our brain function—whether that means to eliminate middle-aged brain fog, think more clearly in meetings, focus attention more sharply, improve brain (and by extension, physical) performance, or simply build a better and stronger brain to sustain us as we age—to learn a little bit about the structure of the brain and how it operates. Don't worry; it's not going to get too technical. You don't have to be a brain surgeon to understand this; just stick with me for the high points.

This Is Your Brain 101

Let's start inside and work our way out. A brain is made up of an enormous number of individual cells—hundreds of billions of them—consisting of four basic types: *neurons*, the ones designed to process information; *astrocytes*, star-shaped cells that provide both physical and metabolic support to the neurons, which they outnumber 10 to 1; *oligodendrocytes,* which produce a type of fatty insulation, called myelin, that coats the interconnections or wiring between brain cells to cut down on static and speed electrical transmission; and *microglia*, the brain's trash collectors or clean-up crew that, much like white blood cells in the body, patrol their domain on the look out for anything that doesn't belong there, such as a germ, a foreign substance, blood outside the blood vessels, or the debris of damaged or worn-out cells or cell parts. Let's take a moment to look a little more closely at how these cells work.

THE NEURONS

Throughout this book, when I use the term *brain cell* I am in most cases referring to neurons, the special cells of the brain designed to relay the information that allows us to move, to talk, to remember, and to perceive and understand the things we can hear, see, touch, smell, and taste in the world around us.

The neuron's shape favors its relay function: It has a body, which houses all the encoded genetic information that controls the cell as well as some of the energy-production equipment. Extensions of a sort project from either side; the vast bulk of the neuron's energy production equipment lies at the ends of these extensions, where most of the energy-intensive activity occurs. The neuron cell bodies and their nearby local connections make up what is called the *gray matter*, and the far-reaching connections (covered with the myelin insulation) make up what's called *white matter*.

From one side of the neuron, the longer of these extensions—called the *axon*—projects out to meet the next neuron. Its length may be measured in microscopically small dimensions for local connections within the brain or may be several feet long, reaching all the way from the cell's body, which lies in either the brain or the spinal cord, to the tips of the fingers or toes. When you cut a nerve, for instance, in your foot, knee, or hand, what you're cutting are bundles of possibly thousands of these myelin-coated extensions, each one of which is a part of an individual neuron with a cell body a very long way away. Amazing, isn't it?

At the other end of the neuron is a cluster of (usually) shorter extensions, called the *dendrites*, which make up the last element of the relay design; they're responsible for collecting incoming information. The relay system is set up by connecting neurons end to end with one another—that is, the axon of one neuron meets the dendrites of another neuron, which connects via its axon to the dendrites of other neurons, and on and on. These complex interconnections (incredibly, a single neuron may receive input from as many as 10,000 others) allow brain signals to travel rapidly to all required areas of the brain virtually simultaneously.

Even more amazing, despite transmissions going nearly everywhere at once, an electrical signal flows only one way in the neuron relay, from the dendrites that receive the signal, through the cell body, and then along its axon to the dendrites of other neurons. This vast interconnectivity isn't actually a physical one; the axon of one neuron doesn't really connect with the dendrites of its neighbors. Although they lie very close, a tiny gap, called the *synaptic cleft*, separates them. When the electrical signal reaches the end of an axon, it causes the release of specific chemical messengers, called *neurotransmitters*, some of which may already be familiar to you: norepinephrine, dopamine, acetylcholine, serotonin, γ-aminobutyric acid (GABA), glutamate, and many more. These neurotransmitters float across the gap, where each docks on the far side into a slot expressly fitted to its shape (called a receptor) and where it passes the information to the next neuron, stimulating yet another electrical wave that whizzes through that neuron's body and down its axon to the synaptic cleft, and so on. The submicroscopic area where the axon endings of one neuron meet the dendrite fibers of the next, including the space that separates them, is called a *synapse*, which is really where the rubber meets the road in brain function. You will learn much more about that and why it is so important later in the chapter.

After each electrical wave passes through it, the neuron must reset itself. It does so by actively pumping such chemical substances as calcium, magnesium, potassium, and sodium back across its outermost layer, called the *cell membrane*. This resetting activity—one of the most energy-gobbling processes in the body—occurs repeatedly, sometimes hundreds or even thousands of times each second, and is in large measure responsible for the high energy demands of the brain.

These synapses or interconnections between the neurons are not fixed like the wiring of a house, but rather change repeatedly throughout our lives, forming anew as we perceive, respond, and experience or regressing with disuse. This phenomenon, called *plasticity*, is what allows us to learn and is in great measure what accounts for much of what makes us human. However, at the same time, it makes the brain exquisitely vulnerable to damage. That's also a topic you'll learn more about later in this chapter.

BRAIN ANATOMY

All these billions of brain cells group together into hundreds of clusters, called nuclei or regions, based generally on their main function—for instance, a cluster of brain cells in the back of the head controls your vision; a grouping on the left side of your head, above your ears, controls language; a pair of nuclei are intimately involved in memory; other clusters control emotion, hearing, the perception of odors, the movement of hands, fingers, toes, or the ability of the skin of your cheek to feel a light touch or the prick of a pin. The brain is just the assembly of these various regions into a single organ. Here's how it all came together as the brain evolved from its very simplest origins in creatures living some 500 million years ago to the exquisitely complex organ that is the modern human brain.

At the base of the brain, just where the spinal cord enters the skull, sits a

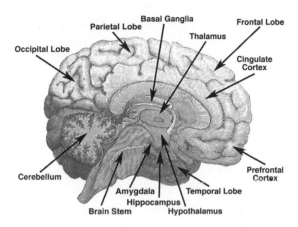

Figure1: View of the medial (inner) surface of the brain

collection of brain cells called the *brain stem* (see Figure 1). This tiny struc-ture, about the size of your little finger, contains a number of clusters of nerve cells that control such basic functions as telling us to breathe, to go to sleep, and to wake up. The parts of the brain that control heartbeat, balance, movement of the eyes, and functions such as coughing and swallowing also reside primarily in the brain stem. Also housed here are networks of cells re-sponsible for alerting distant centers of higher brain function that their ac-tions might be necessary. All in all, many vital survival functions are densely packed into this small space.

Sitting atop the brain stem rests another primitive assemblage of gray matter nuclei of ancient origin, called the *thalamus*, *hypothalamus*, and *basal ganglia*. I say "primitive," because these structures have been around nearly as long as there have been rudimentary brains of almost any sort. For eons, they have guided the behavior of reptiles and some birds, which don't pos-sess a higher, thinking brain.

Although they are neighbors in this region, these structures serve very different—although related—functions. The thalamus receives and processes the incoming sensory information from the world around us. The basal gan-glia act on what the thalamus learns about the outside world and direct any body movements they deem necessary based on that information. Just as the thalamus monitors the external world, the hypothalamus monitors what's going on inside and acts to keep it in balance, regulating such functions as appetite, body temperature, thirst, hormone activity, and our response to stress.

Sitting at the lower back of the brain is the *cerebellum*, a brain region about the size of a lemon. Brain signals from the cerebellum influence coordination; balance; the stability of the trunk of the body; and the fine muscle control needed for such activities as writing, painting, and playing the piano.

The brain continued to evolve over the millennia in response to increased information processing demands. For example, as finding food or eluding predators became more and more complex, the need arose for higher centers of thinking. Among the first steps in that direction was the development of another ancient part of the brain known as the *limbic system*, which controls emotional traits, such as fear, anxiety, and anger as well as memory and spatial navigation. After all, knowing the best route to the nearest water hole and recalling where the den of lions is located along the way have definite survival value. Three brain structures contribute to the make up of the limbic system: the *hippocampus*, which plays a pivotal role in memory; the *cingulate cortex*, which is involved in ranking the importance of events that befall us with an eye toward how they might affect us and whether we need to pay attention and/or worry; and the *amygdala*, which is involved in the processing and interpretation of emotionally charged states such as aggression and fear.

The most recent expansion in the evolution of the brain—called the *neocortex*, meaning "new cortex"—is the familiar layer of wrinkled gray hills and valleys visible on the brain's surface. This structure, which makes up the lion's share of the higher brain or the cortex, is present only in mammals and is highly developed in humans. The neocortex is an intricately folded sheet of brain cells and connections just a few millimeters thick that when unfolded would cover 200,000 square millimeters. This compact, tightly folded form reduces the amount of wiring needed to connect the various regions. Compared to the lower centers of the brain, the neocortex is much more richly wired. Moreover, the circuitry here is highly plastic, by which I mean it's con-

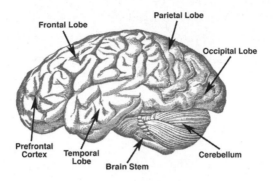

Figure 2: View of the lateral (outside) surface of the brain

tinuously rewiring itself in response to what we experience, much like having a computer that is able to upgrade its hardware continuously without the need for direction or down time. Plasticity, however, comes at a price: the highly plastic brain is also highly vulnerable to damage.

The neocortex has four distinct regions, called lobes, that each generally perform a particular function (see Figure 2). For instance, the *occipital lobe*, located in the back of the brain, allows us to see by interpreting the sensory information our eyes collect. The *frontal lobe*, the front half of the brain located behind the forehead, takes charge of planning and executing the actions of our muscles. In the very front of the frontal lobe lies an area called the *prefrontal cortex* (PFC), once called the "silent brain" because it didn't seem to do anything or at least no one understood what it did. The PFC is now recognized as the seat of executive functions; it's the part of our brain that allows us to imagine a future we've never seen based on a learned and remembered past and to create a mental image about what we'd like to do and design a program for bringing that desired action into being.

Working sort of like the CEO of a company or the conductor of an orchestra, the PFC devises an overall game plan toward a specific goal or purpose and then delegates and directs the jobs that need to be done to accomplish that task to the regions of the brain best suited to doing the job; for this reason, the prefrontal area is the most highly wired part of the brain, densely and directly connected to every other functional region. This arrangement allows for an efficient and highly flexible thinking and reacting machine. The downside, however, is that the very richness of interconnections that makes it so flexible also renders the neocortex in general (and the PFC in particular) more vulnerable to disease, damage, and degeneration with age than any other part of the brain. It's like a high-performance engine; it runs great when it's well maintained but sputters and chokes when it's neglected.

On either side of the brain, just above the ear, sit the *temporal lobes*, which handle the processing of sound and, in the case of mainly the left temporal lobe, of speech and language. This lopsided location of the speech center in the brain is why people who suffer a stroke on the left side of the brain experience greater problems with speech than those who have a stroke on the right side.

Just above the temporal areas, higher on the sides of the brain, lie the *parietal lobes*, which deal with processing of complex sensory messages, especially those dealing with our tactile senses, meaning those involving the sense of touch. These areas allow us to perceive the difference between the pleasure of feeling beach sand between our toes versus the discomfort of the same sand in our sandals chaffing those same toes.

None of these higher brain activities would work, however, if not for neurotransmitters, those brain chemical messengers that shoot the gap of the synapse to convey information from neuron to neuron. Let's take a look at a few of them.

THE NEUROTRANSMITTERS

Neurotransmitters are small chemical compounds that act in the brain as the messengers through which one neuron talks to another. Like the shouting traders on the stock exchange floor, all clamoring that their message be heard, neurotransmitters flood the trillions of synapses throughout the brain hundreds or thousands of times a second, at any given time with some shouting more loudly than others. For instance, the neurotransmitter *glutamate* speaks a message that excites the neurons; it is opposed by the message of

GABA, which has a calming effect. These two neurotransmitters exert an opposite yin–yang or on–off effect directly on individual neurons; others work more subtly, gently adjusting the volume control of messages involving large groups of neurons. What the brain hears depends on the balance between them all. In the following paragraphs, I discuss some of the major neurotransmitters and the roles they play.

Acetylcholine (ACH), the first neurotransmitter to be identified, acts in the body to regulate a broad array of what are called *autonomic functions*, such as regulating heart rate, blood pressure, glandular functions, and the motions of the intestinal tract. In the brain, however, ACH is chiefly involved in the storage and retrieval of learned (remembered) information. A shortage of it—such as occurs in Alzheimer's disease—impairs memory, making it difficult to find a word, to balance a checkbook, or to recall a name or face. Supplements or medications that let ACH linger within the synapse just a brief moment longer can substantially improve memory, which is the way that drugs, such as Aricept work

Dopamine (DA), keenly involved in such brain functions as attention and focus, is also necessary for smooth coordinated movements. It is probably best known as a major player in Parkinson's disease, the devastating neurodegenerative disorder that afflicts over half a million Americans, including celebrities Michael J. Fox and Muhammad Ali. Research implicates a lack of dopamine signaling in the symptoms of Parkinson's, accounting for the flatness of facial expression, the shuffling gait, the uncoordinated and jerky motions, and the shaking tremors that are the hallmarks of the disease. Restoring dopamine action with medications is one of the most successful treatments for the disorder.

Norepinephrine (NE) keeps tabs on our internal environment; regulates our body temperature, metabolic rate, and appetite; releases many hormones, and oversees our emergency readiness to fight or run when danger threatens.

Serotonin, or more correctly the lack of it, has become widely known as a cause for depression and the basis for an entire class of antidepressant drugs, the so-called selective serotonin reuptake inhibitors (SSRIs) typified by Prozac. Serotonin is a feel-good neurotransmitter that sends messages involved in regulation of social and emotional areas, including mood, anxiety, and fear. Proper serotonin balance also improves sleep.

Taurine, which is an amino acid that behaves much like a neurotransmitter, is involved in adjusting the volume on inflammation signals that arise from such things as trauma or ischemia (loss of blood supply to an area) or in circumstances when nerve cells are overstimulated, such as in states of excitotoxicity.

Although these are only a few of the scores of compounds that can transmit signals within the brain, they are the group most pertinent to the scope of this book and this brief discussion should sufficiently serve to acquaint you with the basic concept. I'd now like to shift gears to look at yet another type of brain cell, one that can be intimately involved in the decline of memory as we age.

THE MICROGLIA

I mentioned earlier that microglia serve a function in the brain similar to the infection-fighting white blood cells in the rest of the body. They move throughout the brain keeping house, picking up and recycling bits of debris, culling old worn-out cells, and sweeping out anything that doesn't belong. But they're not merely the brain's janitorial crew; they're also like drug-sniffing dogs, trained to detect the chemical "odor" of foreign invaders, objects, or substances that might be dangerous to the brain and to attack and destroy them if necessary. They can also spot danger in other ways—for instance, by detecting the special chemicals a neuron releases when it's stressed physically or metabolically. When the microglia identify an invader or a distress signal, they sound an alarm that triggers a cascade of inflammation designed to neutralize the problem, which often means destroying whatever is causing it.

This SWAT team function of the microglia, just as for their white blood cell cousins, is an ancient defense mechanism designed to turn on, identify and handle the problem, and promptly turn off once the danger has been dealt with or has passed. Sometimes, however, the panic button gets stuck in the on position, which keeps the microglia in full SWAT mode and sets up escalating cycles of inflammation that can extensively damage the brain. This kind of inappropriate long-term inflammatory alert is what goes awry in such progressive, destructive, and disabling brain disorders as multiple sclerosis (MS).[1] Especially important for our discussion, chronic activation of the microglia, although to a far milder degree, is also a part of what happens in the aging brain that robs us of our mental capabilities and memory. On that score, let's take a moment in our survey of how the brain is put together to look at how memory works.

Memory at Work

Have you ever seen a photograph of an old-time telephone switchboard? A bank of operators sat in a row (in big cities there would be entire rooms of them) each in front of a switchboard awash with blinking lights and crisscrossing networks of wires through which she (and it usually was a *she*) connected one phone caller to another. Although on an infinitely more complex scale, that's pretty much how neurons talk to one another: One hooks up to another one—or actually about 10,000 other ones—for a chat. The depth and breadth of the brain's switchboard becomes clear when you understand that a single human brain sends more communication signals in a day than all the telephones in the world. With all these signals zinging through the wiring, how is it that we can think and remember and act in an orderly fashion? How does the mind work?

At birth, except for the primitive parts of the brain that we need for survival—the brain stem and the limbic system—we begin with a brain switchboard that is mostly blank. The higher brain centers, including the frontal lobes and prefrontal cortex, mature rather late in development, because the trillions

---

1. In MS, the immune system (including the microglia) attacks and destroys sections of the myelin insulation in the brain and around nerves, which paves the way for the electrical static, slower transmission, short-circuiting, and loss of signals that give rise to the unpredictable bouts of symptoms—such as numbness, tingling, sudden loss of control of a limb or of vision—that are the hallmarks of the disease. The underlying cause of the autoimmune attack is as yet unsettled.

of hookups (the synapses) located there must be connected, reconnected, and sculpted by early life experiences. Connecting the switchboard comes at a huge energy cost; the newborn human infant's brain gobbles up almost two-thirds of the energy used by its entire body, whereas the adult brain demands only about 20 percent of the body's energy production. That amount still makes it king of the hill in the body's energy-use sweepstakes, but it pales next to the energy requirement of an infant brain busily wiring and rewiring all its circuits.

Each new learning experience for a brain of any age stimulates a new hookup. Repetition solidifies the hookup and triggers the brain to make it semipermanent by coating the connections in myelin, sort of like soldering speaker wires in place in your audio system versus loosely twisting them together. It makes for less static and a surer, faster connection, so that we can call learned information back up more easily and quickly at some future time, sometimes even automatically.

What we call *memory* is the process by which the brain retains learned experiences over time through these physical, hardwired synapse connections. Scientists divide the memory files along two basic lines. The first is *procedural* memory, which relates to the learning of a task or skill, such as typing, playing the piano, walking, riding a bike, or roller skating—that is, a procedure, the performance of which can be improved by practice until it becomes quite automatic. The second basic kind of memory file, *declarative* memory, involves the storage of facts, such things as your phone number or address, the names of your grandchildren, all the U.S. presidents, or who conquered England in 1066.

Declarative memory itself further divides into two distinct areas. The first of these is called *semantic* memory, which includes the storage of learned facts and concepts. It's, for the most part, the kind of memory we rely on in school to learn the three *R*s (reading, 'riting, and 'rithmetic) and is subject to forgetting without regular repetition to keep the circuits fresh.

The second kind, termed *episodic* memory, involves your personal recollection of events and the times, places, and emotions surrounding them. In general, the more emotion tied to an event, the stronger and more vivid the episodic memory for it. For instance, if you were alive in 1963, you can likely answer this question without hesitation: Where were you when you learned President Kennedy had been shot? Watershed events, such as this one, produce what's been called *flashbulb memory*, meaning that the event almost instantly generates lasting interconnections between brain cells. The storage vault for flashbulb memory, as is the case for all declarative memories, is primarily through connections within the hippocampus and neocortex. The neuron connections for procedural memory, on the other hand, are mainly in the basal ganglia, cerebellum, and spinal cord.

This physical separation for the two types of memory helps explain why, as we age, we may have trouble calling up the right word or putting a name to a face but can still remember how to ride a bike. The storage areas for declarative memory—the neocortex and hippocampus—because of their high-performance wiring and their need to remain flexible to rewire connections as needed are at much greater risk of degeneration over time. Keeping them functioning optimally for as long as possible—and thus preserving our memory—is our goal. Despite the brain's complexity, understanding what it takes to keep it healthy is actually pretty simple. Every means we might employ to accomplish that goal—whether it's eating a better diet, taking certain brain beneficial nutritional supplements, doing the right kind of exercise, avoiding toxic substances—all work by the effect they have on one or more of just four basic areas that the individual brain cell wants to keep just right.

The Goldilocks Principles

Mathematics is a pure science, very precise: two plus two always equals four, not eight, not seven, not nine. Math is like a standard light switch; it's on or it's off. Biology, on the other hand, isn't at all black and white. To carry the analogy forward, biological processes work more like a rheostat or dimmer switch, for which possible options include on, off, and everywhere in between. As the occasion demands, a given biologic process might be fully turned off, might operate at full-tilt, or might settle at some level in between the two extremes in constant search of the biologic sweet spot that will keep everything clipping happily along.

Although true of the body as a whole, the brain, more than any other or-gan, strives to keep its critical processes operating safely in a "just right" zone as much of the time as possible, not too fast or too slow, not too hot or too cold, not too much or too little. To do so, in the face of the legions of physi-cal, metabolic, chemical, and environmental changes and challenges that oc-cur continuously, the brain must be nimble enough to adjust in fractions of a microsecond. It is interesting that, although the moment-by-moment chal-lenges the brain must handle are nearly limitless, they virtually all involve one or more of only four critical areas that the brain must closely regulate or manage: the flow of calcium, the balance of insulin and glucose (blood sugar), the availability of adequate growth factors for regeneration and re-pair, and the control of inflammation. Virtually every traumatic or toxic in-sult, medication or drug challenge, or change in metabolic or nutritional circumstance presented to the brain affects one or more of these four basic areas, and the brain strives mightily to restore them to the just right balance. For this reason, I call them the brain's *Goldilocks Principles*. To illuminate your understanding of why the brain works as it does; why things go wrong with age, trauma, or illness; and how it's possible to preserve or even improve brain function, let's explore each of the principles in depth.

GOLDILOCKS PRINCIPLE ONE: CONTROLLING THE FLOW OF CALCIUM

Our neurons (or brain cells) must be able to communicate with one another readily for us to perform any of the wondrous activities that make us human. Every action from writing a symphony, singing a song, painting a pic-ture, playing the piano, or chatting with friends to reading a good book or laughing at a joke comes back to the single basic need of neurons to com-municate easily.

Neurons communicate with one another through their synapses, which are outpouchings of their cell membranes (or skins) that form the points of contact between them and their neighbors. (In a very simplistic sense, you can think of the synapses as being sort of like the tin cans on the ends of string that kids use to talk to one another.) However, the system is extraordinarily complex, in that each and every neuron receives incoming communication (that is, a synaptic contact point) from as many as 10,000 other neurons. When you factor in that there are approximately 100 billion neurons in the human brain, it means that the average brain contains 1,000 trillion contact points continuously firing, continuously communicating with one another.

Unlike the analogy of the tin can, however, synapses aren't fixed in shape or location; they emerge, regress, rewire, and reshape, quite literally hour by hour, under the continuous sculpting influence of our history (past knowledge or activity) and the incoming load of new information. We call this real-time reshaping of synapses *plasticity*, and it is the basis for all learning, memory, attention, and emotion—in short, for our humanity.

A good way to think about synapse formation is to liken it to the raising of a circus tent. The workers initially spread the large canvas out on the ground, then, going beneath it, they begin to raise parts of it with telescoping poles. Gradually, the dome appears; and then, as the workers tighten the ropes, the full canopy emerges.

The raising of a new synapse occurs in much the same way. A small area of the brain cell membrane represents the canvas, which is raised from the surface by the construction of microtubules inside the cell, submicroscopic in size—the tiny tent poles, if you will. The poles of this synaptic scaffolding fit tightly one to the next, end to end, lashed together by binding proteins, called *tau* proteins. (Remember this term because tau proteins play a major role in memory loss, especially in Alzheimer's disease.)

But where, you may ask, does calcium figure in? It is the precisely coordinated and regulated flow of calcium ions into the cell that triggers both the construction of the tubules and their lashing together via the tau proteins, meaning that all learning, memory, attention, and emotion ultimately depend on the brain's being able to control calcium inflow flawlessly.[2] And control

---

2. Although calcium is the workhorse of nerve cell communication, its release depends on yet another brain chemical, called glutamate, a chemical found in foods (the flavor enhancer monosodium glutamate, MSG, for example) that in substantial amounts can be brain toxic, more about which later.

calcium it must, since true to its Goldilocks nature, the amount of calcium in the cell can't be too little or too much, but just right. The cell allows the calcium to flow in on cue and do its business, then expends tremendous energy to shove the calcium back out, because allowing it to build up inside the cell is potentially lethal. With too little calcium, the synapse won't become excited enough to fire it's signal; with too much, the nerve cell will literally excite itself to death.

Deviation of calcium concentrations much outside the just right zone can disrupt the balance between the raising and tearing down of synapses. When excess tearing down occurs the neurons become disconnected, which impairs brain function. It's what happens to a degree in the memory loss of aging and, at its extreme, is what happens in Alzheimer's disease.

GOLDILOCKS PRINCIPLE TWO: CONTROLLING THE BALANCE OF INSULIN AND GLUCOSE

The brain has a sweet tooth; it demands a continuous diet of glucose (blood sugar) as its main fuel source, removing roughly 100 grams (about ½ cup) of it from the blood each day to keep its synapses humming along. That's not an amount too hard to come by in our age of carbohydrate-heavy foods, such as bagels and pasta, but our biochemical machinery didn't arise in the land of carb plenty. Rather, we evolved mainly eating meat and supplementing that by gathering whatever meager carb resources nature seasonally offered, which in some climes might have been minimal. So how did our early ancestors fulfill the brain's glucose demands? The answer—biochemically.

Their brains, like ours, needed a daily sugar fix. To meet these needs, the human body is ingeniously equipped to produce all the glucose the brain requires from protein. The protein comes either from what we consume in our diets or, in times of outright starvation—since the body can store enough sugar to last only about 24 hours before trouble starts—from dipping into the body's protein reservoir (the muscles, bones, and other organs) for raw materials that the body can turn into glucose.

With plenty of protein and fat to eat and all things biochemical working normally, both brain and body can do quite nicely for the long haul on a diet with limited sources of carbohydrates. It's what we cut our teeth on evolutionarily speaking.

Fair enough, but where, you might wonder, does insulin come in? After all, insulin is a hormone we associate with diabetes, with bringing blood sugar down when it's too high. And indeed that is true. When we eat a meal, our digestive processes break the food into proteins, fats, and sugars. The proteins and sugars inspire the body to release insulin, which acts to drive these two nutrients out of the blood and into the tissues where they can be used. This natural human feeding cycle works just fine, so long as we have access to food, either to glucose or something, such as protein, that we can turn into glucose.

Somewhere along the way, our bodies learned a clever trick to help meet the brain's need for glucose in times of want; we developed the ability to render ourselves temporarily insulin resistant. To better understand what this means to the body or brain, think of insulin as the key that opens the door through which the glucose can leave the blood and enter the muscles or other tissues; insulin resistance, then, acts to jam the lock, making the key ineffective and slamming the door shut to the passage of glucose.

The muscles, organs, and even the heart can operate quite well (even prefer to operate) on fat as a fuel source for energy production. By becoming temporarily insulin resistant, the muscles and organs turn to fat burning for energy, which preserves all the glucose in the blood for the sugar-addicted brain.[3] When food becomes plentiful again, our bodies return to a state of normal insulin sensitivity, and all is again right with the world. So from an evolutionary perspective, because periods of starvation usually didn't last too long, being able to render ourselves transiently insulin resistant served us well by making us better able to survive lean times.

Now fast-forward to the present, when at least in the affluent West there is rarely any lack of carbohydrates or calories. It would seem logical that under

3. Transient insulin resistance also occurs in women during the last few months of pregnancy, when the mother's blood sugar must be divided between two brains—hers and her baby's. The condition usually resolves after delivery. In some women, it occurs to the degree that frank diabetes ensues, which sometimes fails to resolve after delivery.

such circumstances, the brain would function optimally, happily bathed in a never-ending sea of blood sugar. However, quite the opposite is true. Although our bodies evolved the machinery to save us from want, times of plenty have been so relatively brief in the course of human history that we haven't developed any means of coping with the reverse. Starvation produces insulin resistance (to preserve brain function under adverse conditions), so almost counterintuitively does consumption of too many calories. Chronic intake of far too much of the wrong foods has saddled some 30 million of us, adults and children alike, with insulin resistance or frank diabetes. For these people, a temporary survival trick has been subverted into a way of life in which both insulin levels and glucose levels run high all the time, creating the metabolic paradox for body and brain of starving in the face of plenty. All the blood sugar in the world can't fuel a brain resistant to insulin. And there are dire and damaging consequences to having too much of either insulin or glucose.

Apart from controlling blood sugar (or not, as in the case of insulin resistance) does insulin play a role in the brain? Until not so long ago, the answer of the medical community would have been a resounding no. But that all changed recently when researchers discovered the presence of insulin receptors in many regions of the brain—and it is interesting that they are in the brain centers controlling appetite, complex thinking, and memory. Insulin itself has also been found in the brain and the big question now is what exactly is it there to do? Clearly, in the appetite center it acts as it does in the muscles, opening the door for the entry of glucose into the brain cells. In other areas, its role isn't so obvious. One intriguing bit of research gives us some clues, however.

Divining what a hormone or body chemical does isn't always straightforward; in fact, it's often easier to see what a substance does by getting rid of it and observing what *doesn't* happen. That's just what a group of researchers did with a strain of mice that have been bred to lack insulin receptors in their brains. The scientists noted that the brains of these mice weren't able to use glucose as well as their normal counterparts. That's not so surprising, but what did get the researchers' attention is that the mice also developed unusual changes in their brains that were quite similar to what is seen in the brains of humans who have Alzheimer's disease. Moreover, the mice not only lost important memory functions, which hampered their ability to find their way through a maze, they also displayed demented behavior. All these findings are analogous to the changes seen in Alzheimer's disease in humans. At least in the case of the mice, the symptoms stemmed entirely from the brain's no longer being able to maintain glucose and insulin in balance. From this observation (and others like it) the second Goldilocks Principle arises: an inability of the body to become insulin resistant is deadly to the brain in the face of starvation; chronic insulin resistance is deadly in the face of overabundance. Once again, the brain wants it to be just right.

GOLDILOCKS PRINCIPLE THREE: CONTROLLING GROWTH, REGENERATION, AND REPAIR

Within the mother's womb, an unborn baby grows from a single cell into a fully formed newborn in a 9-months-long biologic ballet directed by growth factors, which are microhormone messengers that stimulate, regulate, and orchestrate the production and maintenance of new cells. The infant grows into a toddler, the toddler into an adolescent, the adolescent into a teen, the teen into an adult, all under the influence of specific growth factors. From before birth and throughout adult life, growth factors direct the building, remodeling, and repair of the entire body, including the brain.

Scientists once believed that we were born with a complete complement of all the brain cells we would ever have and that we began the process of losing them from that time on. Extremely exciting new research has now proven it's possible for the mature adult brain to form new brain cells capable of connecting and integrating into existing communication networks, so long as our brain can maintain an adequate supply of certain vital growth factors. (Most intriguing of all, we can diminish or replenish the supply with the lifestyle choices we make!)

At birth, a newborn brain contains many more neurons than it will eventually have as an adult. In fact, in infancy, the number of synapses peaks at about double the adult number. Why should this be, considering that infants are clearly smaller and less capable than adults and, one would assume, far less in need of a rich network of connections? The answer lies in the phenomenon of *plasticity*, the ever-changing ability of the human brain to reshape its connections in order to learn and remember.

From the moment we are born, and even before, our brains begin to process enormous amounts of incoming sensory information—the cold air, the bright light, the pain of needlesticks, the sound of voices, the warmth of a parent's arms. Each sensory input throughout life, but especially so in our earliest formative years, works like a tiny chisel, sculpting the brain; solidifying new skills, new data, new faces, and new places; strengthening oft-used connections; and pruning away redundant and unused ones. And that's where the huge excess of an infant's neurons and synapses comes into play; it allows for plenty of raw material for the individual human experience to sculpt into a mature, adult brain with its vast networks of interconnected, rapidly communicating brain cells in what amounts to survival of the most connected. Neurons were born to communicate. Those that do so successfully become integrated into fully functional communication circuits that allow us to remember a fact; a face; and how to walk, talk, or smile. Those that fail to form solid connections based on our exposures and experiences get weeded out.

The process of connecting neurons to one another, which results in our ability to remember and to learn, progresses in stages as we grow, fueled by what seems like a veritable alphabet soup of growth promoters: nerve growth factor (NGF), neurotrophin 3 (NT3), and brain-derived neurotrophic factor (BDNF) among them. BDNF, for instance, supports the growth and survival of new brain cells; increases their resistance to injury; and spurs the construction, remodeling, and rewiring of new synapses or connections between brain cells from before birth to death. And, as experimental work with mice deficient in BDNF has shown, lack of it impairs learning and memory. It is interesting that some human research indicates that the lack of BDNF can be true a deficiency (not enough BDNF present) or merely a functional one—in other words, a resistance can develop to BDNF, not unlike the resistance our muscles can develop to insulin, in which there's plenty of it around, but the cells are blind to its message.

Fluidity of thought depends on uninterrupted, high-speed communication among the interconnected brain cells. If the connection is spotty, the brain cells can process and react to only a fraction of the incoming information. If these regions become functionally disconnected, it's like being dropped from a conference call. Specialized brain-scanning technology has demonstrated the loss of functional connectivity with age, a finding that correlates with an age-related decline in ability to perform certain tasks.

The brain relies on growth factors, such as BDNF, to maintain the balance between making new connections among brain cells (or strengthening existing ones) and weeding out or pruning them away. Loss of BDNF support (whether through lack of its production or blunting of its message) tips the balance toward pruning connections and loss of brain cells. Once again, the brain strives to keep this process at a just right level; if it cannot, brain function suffers. The good news for us all is that we can, through the lifestyle choices recommended in the Brain Trust Program, increase the brain's production of BDNF and tip the balance back in our favor.

GOLDILOCKS PRINCIPLE FOUR: CONTROLLING INFLAMMATION

In first-century C.E. Rome, Celsus described inflammation as having four classic signs: swelling, redness, pain, and warmth, or in the Latin, *tumor*, *rubor*, *dolor*, and *calor*. In the intervening millennia, we haven't really been able to improve on his description of the outward and visible signs of the inflammatory response. His four *-ors,* taught to this day in medical schools around the world, still offer a perfect picture of what we can see and feel when something incites such a response: think infected splinter, mosquito bite, pink eye, or appendicitis. The misery occasioned by these conditions stems chiefly from the body's highly specific assault against something it perceives as a foreign enemy and its effort to drive it out by unleashing the only weapon at its command: the immune system.

We depend on a highly vigilant immune system both to protect us from attack by the bacteria, viruses, and fungi in the world around us and to recognize and eliminate any rogue cells that arise within; cells that left unchecked could form cancers. For instance, if you step on a rusty nail, the puncture will carry whatever bacteria might have been on the nail or the sole of your bare foot into the depth of the wound. The trauma itself causes the release of special inflammatory compounds, chemical signals that, like an SOS, will draw the immune system's advance force of white blood cells into the area to survey the situation and, through the release of inflammatory compounds of their own, call up the appropriate reinforcements required to attack and destroy whatever isn't supposed to be there and to clean up the mess on the field of battle afterward.

Natural selection fashioned the immune system to be on constant watch, to respond swiftly and powerfully to specific insults of limited duration when called on to do so, and to stand down once the enemy had been defeated. The system isn't so well suited, however, to being constantly stimulated and chronically deployed. The development of such diseases as rheumatoid arthritis and MS offer vivid examples of the damage wrought when a chronically stimulated immune system turns on itself. Within the body, inflammation has a vital role, but it must be controlled. The same applies to the brain.

Instead of the white blood cell brigade that patrols the body, the brain relies on microglia to be on the lookout for and fight the battles against microbes and other invaders as well as to handle the business of cleaning up cellular debris and recycling the junk proteins and other detritus that accumulate from living. Like the white blood cells, the microglia also respond to the call of inflammatory compounds.

As the brain ages, it loses volume and weight as the number of neurons and connections between neurons dwindles. It is surprising that, at the same time, the number of microglia actually appears to increase and, with them, the levels of the inflammatory compounds they make and release.

Although modern science hasn't been able to improve on the outward description of inflammation that Celsus offered two millennia ago, it's done yeoman's work in describing and helping us understand what goes on at a microscopic, submicroscopic, and even chemical level. Those inflammatory compounds that the white blood cells and microglia release into the locale of a perceived enemy are a good example. One, in particular, called tumor necrosis factor α (TNFα), has critical relevance for the brain: TNFα interferes with the action of BDNF, the loss of which as you've already learned impairs memory, reaction speed, and facile thinking. As levels of TNFα rise and BDNF activity falls, the brain becomes less able to create and repair synaptic connections and less able to withstand the stress from toxins, excess calcium, and injuries.

What would make the levels of TNFα rise? Examples include insulin resistance and/or diabetes, which makes controlling that system of added importance. In a cyclic cascade of unfortunate events, excess blood sugar leads to elevated insulin; which leads to insulin resistance; which is associated with excess TNFα; which leads to resistance to BDNF's message; which leads to a net loss of functional brain cell connections; which, finally, leads to memory decline, slowed reaction speed, and depressed mood, among other things.

In keeping with the Goldilocks directive, the inflammatory response team within the brain must be vigilant and engaged, but not overstimulated.

The three pillars of the Brain Trust Program—nutrition, supplementation, and exercise for the body and brain—work in concert to maintain the just right balance in each of the four Goldilocks Principles. And for this reason, I encourage you to work the program in its entirety for best results.

3

Are You at Risk?

Knowing that a brain problem may exist or being aware of ways to prevent it has no value unless you can reliably determine whether or not you should care. Where do *you* fall on the spectrum of memory, organization, and focus abilities? Are you as sharp as you used to be or as you'd like to be? Are you able to remain vigilant for long periods while performing tedious work or do you notice your attention wandering? Is it easy for you to concentrate on mental tasks such as reading or do you find yourself having to go over paragraphs or sentences again and again because of brain fog? Are you at greater risk for memory decline because of family history, medical status, or lifestyle? Many such factors can affect brain health.

In this chapter, you will learn about these risk factors in detail, what they are and how they work to rob us of our memory or slow our thought processes and reflexes. In subsequent chapters, you'll also learn the good news about effective remedies and recommendations to circumvent such problems.

Before we get into that discussion, however, I'd like you to take stock of your own situation by answering a series of pertinent questions that will help you pinpoint where you (or someone you love) falls on the spectrum of brain health.

BRAIN RISK ASSESSMENT QUESTIONNAIRE

PART 1

You should answer each of the following questions with the number that best describes you. Feel free to make a copy of these pages to use in answering the questions. Scoring is from 0 to 3 for each response. You may find it helpful and enlightening for another person who knows you well to independently answer these questions about you and then compare your responses.

0	1	2	3
Never	Rarely	Occasionally	Frequently

Answers		
Others	Yours	
_____	_____	1. Do you misplace things (like keys, glasses, wallet)?
_____	_____	2. Do you have trouble finding the right word?
_____	_____	3. Must you write things down so you don't forget to do them?
_____	_____	4. Do you have poor attention to details?
_____	_____	5. Are you easily distracted?
_____	_____	6. Are you impulsive, acting before thinking?
_____	_____	7. If the radio or TV is on, do you have difficulty concentrating?
_____	_____	8. If interrupted, is it difficult to remember where you left off?
_____	_____	9. Do you forget your train of thought while speaking?
_____	_____	10. Do you have increased difficulty with mental calculations (like computing a tip, balancing a checkbook)?
_____	_____	11. Are new tasks more difficult to learn than you previously experienced (using a DVD player, VCR, or computer, for instance)?

_____ _____ 12. Do you find it increasingly difficult to follow movie plots?

_____ _____ 13. Do you have feelings of unexplained sadness?

_____ _____ 14. Do you have feelings of unexplained nervousness?

_____ _____ 15. Do you suffer from low self-esteem?

_____ _____ 16. Have you withdrawn from friends and social activities?

_____ _____ 17. Do you have feelings of panic, fear, or anxiety for no apparent reason?

_____ _____ 18. Are there major stresses in your life (work, money, family)?

_____ _____ 19. Have you been required to contend with prior stressful situations (wartime, childhood abuse, death/loss)?

_____ _____ 20. Must you deal with major illnesses (or those of a parent, sibling, or child)?

PART 2

Yes   No

_____ _____ 21. Do you have a parent, grandparent, or sibling who has suffered from Alzheimer's disease, dementia, or has had a stroke?

_____ _____ 22. Do you have type 1 or type 2 diabetes?

_____ _____ 23. Do you have coronary artery disease?

_____ _____ 24. Do you have blood pressure with a systolic reading (higher number) greater than 140 or diastolic (lower number) greater than 80?

_____ _____ 25. Have you ever been diagnosed with depression?

_____ _____ 26. Have you ever been diagnosed with post-traumatic stress disorder (PTSD)?

_____ _____ 27. Have you ever had a head injury resulting in loss of consciousness?

_____ _____ 28. Are you more than 30 pounds overweight?

_____ _____ 29. Do you exercise less than 3 hours per week? (Exercise includes walking, swimming, golfing, hiking, dancing, and bike-riding.)

_____ _____ 30. Do you smoke?

_____ _____ 31. Are you a cancer survivor?

_____ _____ 32. Do you eat fatty fish fewer than three times per month? (Fatty fish includes salmon, anchovies, herring, mackerel, and sardines.)

_____	_____	33.	Do you eat trans-fats three or more times per week? (Trans-fats are found in margarine; processed foods such as crackers, cakes, and cookies; Crisco and vegetable shortening; also called partially hydrogenated oils.)
_____	_____	34.	Do you eat deep-fried foods three or more times per week?
_____	_____	35.	Do you routinely get fewer than 6 hours of sleep per night?
_____	_____	36.	Do you have congestive heart failure, emphysema, chronic obstructive pulmonary disease (COPD), or sleep apnea?
_____	_____	37.	Do you use methamphetamines, cocaine, or ecstasy (3, 4-methylenedioxy-methamphetamine; MDMA)?
_____	_____	38.	Do you have, or have you had, periodontal disease with missing or loose teeth?
_____	_____	39.	Do you have osteoporosis?
_____	_____	40.	Do you have elevated homocysteine (greater than or equal to 12)?
_____	_____	41.	Do you drink more than 7 servings (females) or 14 servings (males) of alcohol per week?
_____	_____	42.	Is your head circumference less than 54 centimeters (females) or 56 centimeters (males) *and* have you completed fewer than 16 years of schooling?
_____	_____	43.	Do you have four or more siblings?
_____	_____	44.	Do you watch more than 4 hours of television per day?
_____	_____	45.	Are you over the age of 70?
_____	_____	46.	Do you currently take, or in the past have you taken, oral corticosteroid medications (such as Decadron, prednisone, hydrocortisone, and Medrol) for a prolonged period of time for conditions such as asthma, giant cell arteritis, rheumatoid arthritis, systemic lupus erythematosus (SLE), or any other disorder?

Score 3 points for every yes answer and 0 points for every no answer.

PART 3

Memory Test

For this portion of the test, you'll need paper and pencil and a clock or watch with a second hand (or a kitchen timer) before beginning. The test involves memorizing a list of 10 words during a brief timed interval and then attempting to recall the list after a 20-minute break, so be sure to allot enough time.

Study the following list of words for no more than 1 minute:

pepper

candle

notebook

kayak

umbrella

cabinet

symphony

associate

prosper

bicycle

After your 1-minute period of study, busy yourself with something completely different for 20 minutes: watch TV, read a good book, listen to the radio, chat with a friend, take a walk, write a letter. Be sure to note the time or to set a timer. When time is up, write down each of the words you can remember.

SCORING

12 points for 0 to 3 words

6 points for 4 or 5 words

3 points for 6 or 7 words

0 points for 8 or more words

RISK CATEGORIES

Now, add up the total number of points from the three parts to determine your degree of risk for developing memory impairment with age. Find your score in the following list:

0–15	You are at low risk.
16–30	You are at moderate risk.
31–45	You are at high risk.
Greater than 45	You are at very high risk.

Shortly I'll get into what each of the risk factors of brain health means then address the more complicated issue of how to interpret each of the risk categories to help you make sense of your score. As we delve more deeply into each of the risk factors, you'll immediately see that some of them are clearly more important than others; you may puzzle, however, over why some of them are included at all, seeming on their surface so commonplace that it may hardly make sense to you to call them risk factors. But bear with me; it will became clear.

A Window into Alzheimer's Disease

Before we move on, I'd like to ask you to take an additional test. It will probably appear quite simple, but it poses difficulty for people with even mild dementia. This experience will give you a new degree of insight into the lives of people suffering from Alzheimer's disease and other forms of dementia (or even milder forms of thought and memory problems) and will demonstrate the severity of the mental frustrations they and their caregivers deal with on a daily basis. More important, however, this simple test will bring into stark focus the degree of loss of mental firepower that some of us may face if we don't take good care of our brains.

You may think you'll never perform poorly on this test, but half the people in a crowded room will develop Alzheimer's disease by age 85, and many more will suffer from milder, but still significant, cognitive decline in their 50s, 60s, and 70s.

THE SET TEST
A quick screening test for dementia[1]

For this test, you'll need paper and pencil and a clock or watch with a second hand (or a kitchen timer). Allow 30 seconds per category for the person taking the test to name as many items as possible (maximum 10 per category).

Colors

Animals

Fruits

Towns

Score 1 point for each correct response, for a maximum of 40 points.

TEST RESULTS

Fewer than 15 correct	Likely dementia
15 to 24	Possible dementia
25 and greater	No dementia

This test is fairly straightforward for most people. The scoring spread gives you an indication of how much difficulty a person with a failing or impaired brain has with simple tasks that many of us don't think twice about. Scoring poorly on this simple test doesn't necessarily indicate that a person has Alzheimer's disease or some other form of dementia; a poor score simply highlights the need for further testing and evaluation by a qualified physician.

A clinical diagnosis of dementia includes the following:

- Confirmatory findings on detailed neuropsychological testing

- Deficits in two areas of cognition (for example memory, judgment, or speech)

1. This test is from B. Isaacs and A. T. Kennie. "The Set Test as an Aid to the Detection of Dementia in Old People." *British Journal of Psychiatry* 123 (1973): 467–470.

- Progressive worsening of symptoms

- No alteration in level of consciousness or alertness

- Onset usually after age 65

- Absence of other disorders that could explain the symptoms

If someone you care about demonstrates patterns of abnormal thinking, confusion, personality change, disorientation, speech problems, memory, or any other brain-related sign or symptom—even if that someone is you—consult your health-care provider for further evaluation and diagnosis of potentially treatable conditions. Sometimes, actually quite often, memory difficulties and behavioral changes stem from side effects of prescription or over-the-counter medications or as a consequence of vitamin deficiencies, thyroid problems, drug abuse, depression, or even brain tumors. Only a thorough evaluation can pinpoint the cause, which may or may not be Alzheimer's disease.

What Factors Influence Brain Health and What Puts Your Brain at Risk?

Both our genes and our environment determine the robust quality of our brains at any given instant in our lives. Because it is loss of brain cells and the connections among them that robs us of mental firepower, it stands to reason that the density of those cells and the richness of their interconnections in our mental prime determine our cognitive reserve capacity. In short, the bigger and more wired your brain in early life, the more you can stand to lose and still keep your mental faculties intact in the face of trauma or aging. It should come as no surprise that genes and environment also determine how much of that capacity we will lose over time.

By environment, of course, I don't simply mean the toxic influences from the world around us, but the foods we eat, the supplements we take or don't, the habits we indulge in, the activities (both mental and physical) that we do throughout our lives, and a host of other factors, virtually all of which we can modify if we choose. I'll address each of these areas in turn, but let's look first at the one area that we can't change: our genes.

FAMILY HISTORY

Does a tendency for declining memory with age run in your family? Among your older relatives, has anyone been diagnosed with Alzheimer's disease? If not, that's a good thing, but it doesn't mean you shouldn't still be concerned about brain health. And conversely, if the answer is yes, remember that while the science is pretty clear that having a family history for the diseases of memory increases your risk, inheritance alone doesn't make that risk a certainty. For instance, even if one identical twin develops Alzheimer's disease, as much as half the time, the other twin will not; many other factors are also at work. If you have a positive family history for memory impairment or Alzheimer's disease, it simply makes it even more important that you begin the proper feeding and caring of your brain now.

True inherited Alzheimer's disease is fortunately quite rare, responsible for only about 5 percent of all cases. In this small group of people, memory decline begins much earlier in life, often in the 40s or 50s, and the disease pursues a much more aggressive and rapid course. But a degree of risk can occur even in families in which the genes for true inherited Alzheimer's disease are absent.

The most well documented and much more common example of genetic risk for Alzheimer's disease occurs in people who carry a particular variant of a gene called apolipoprotein E (APOE); we all have the gene for APOE, but about 20 percent of us—one in five people—carry at least one copy of the variant form of the gene that has been associated with increased risk for memory loss.

As is the case with every gene, each of us inherits two copies: one from Mom and the other from Dad. In the case of APOE, each copy can be of one of three types, called epsilon 2, 3, and 4. Only the epsilon 4 (ε4) variety carries with it the risk for developing memory failure. Carrying a single copy of ε4 increases risk of Alzheimer's 4-fold; two copies may increase risk as much as 16-fold.

It's important, however, to understand that genetic testing to determine APOE types, even if your physician were willing to have it done, cannot predict who will develop Alzheimer's disease, because carrying the trait is only a *risk factor*; it doesn't cause the disease to develop. Moreover, even the people who do carry a copy of ε4 could just as well flip a coin to determine their odds: 50 percent of them will and 50 percent will not develop the disease, an odds ratio that once again reminds us that genes don't predict all. When Alzheimer's disease does develop in this group, the onset of symptoms is several decades later than in the true familial pattern, usually beginning in a person's 70s.

Despite its later onset, however, science has uncovered a key early finding. Using positron emission tomography (PET) scanning (a type of specialized scan that can assess metabolic activity), researchers have demonstrated that people in their 30s who carry the ε4 variant of APOE already show abnormalities in glucose metabolism in certain areas of their brains. This important connection offers a potential option to better the odds that APOE ε4 carriers can keep their brains healthy in the face of inherited risk. For this group, and for reasons we'll discuss, controlling insulin and glucose metabolism early in life takes on even greater importance.

The value in knowing this genetic or family information about memory loss lies chiefly in that it points to a heightened need to pay particular attention to the lifestyle choices that can improve (or harm) brain health. Let's delve into that arena now, with a look at what else, besides our genes, may raise or lower our risk for memory or cognitive decline as we age.

INSULIN RESISTANCE, PREDIABETES, AND DIABETES

Research has clearly demonstrated that having elevated blood sugar, diabetes, or insulin resistance increases the risk of developing memory loss with aging—even developing Alzheimer's disease—for all groups, not just for those with the APOE (ε4) gene. Although exactly how diabetes does so isn't clearly understood, the connection between the two is pretty easy to see once you understand that the brain relies primarily on glucose (or blood sugar) to produce the enormous amounts of energy that it needs to do its job. The human brain is quite an energy hog; amazingly, even though it makes up only a few percent of the body's weight, the brain consumes 20 percent of the body's energy production. Under normal circumstances, the brain requires a glucose fix of about 100 grams a day—the equivalent of slightly more than a ½ cup of sugar—to meet its demand for energy. And thus arises its critical dependence on well-oiled blood sugar–regulating machinery.

Poor glucose control in the body means higher glucose presented to the brain. Sustained high glucose levels ultimately lead to persistently elevated insulin, which, in turn, leads to a blunting of the insulin response or insulin resistance, which leads to higher glucose. As the sugar levels increase over time, irreversible chemical reactions begin to occur between the sugar molecules and the proteins in the blood and in the brain, forming substances that science has dubbed *advanced glycation end products*, usually shortened to the highly appropriate acronym AGEs. The attachment of sugar to the proteins not only renders them ineffective but also increases the free-radical burden on the brain, which further damages the brain cells. Clinical research has documented a close association between the buildup of AGEs in the bloodstream with the phenomenon of brain shrinkage. In fact, in one study, the level of AGEs was the single most significant risk factor uncovered for brain shrinkage.

High levels of glucose also trigger elevations of cortisol, which further damages brain cells; disrupts blood sugar metabolism in the brain; and ultimately affects thinking, memory, learning, and reaction speed. I'll delve more deeply into the notion of stress and its effects on the brain a little later on. For now, just keep in mind that high blood sugar plays a role.

Diabetes is also associated with atherosclerosis, which reduces blood flow to the brain, thus robbing it of critical nutrients. This, in turn, makes it that much more difficult for the brain to meet its tremendous energy needs and function at its peak. In addition, the particularly common variant of diabetes associated with obesity (such an intimate association that some researchers have taken to calling the pair *diabesity*) sharply increases inflammation in body and brain.

Studies have shown that an overweight diabetic body is an inflamed body, and new evidence suggests that this inflammation affects the brain, contributing to memory loss and brain shrinkage with age and perhaps playing a role in producing the sticky plaques that are the hallmark of Alzheimer's disease. There may be no more important modifiable risk factor to tackle in the quest for better brain health than diabesity. Toward that end, there's no better place to start than by working on the next risk factor.

EATING A JUNK FOOD DIET

We are, in large part, what we eat, and so it stands to reason that be- cause the brain is especially vulnerable in so many other ways, it would be influenced by the quality of our diet. And so it is. A poor-quality, junk food diet—high in partially hydrogenated vegetable oils, sugar, corn syrup, and other refined carbohydrates—increases the risk of memory loss. For that reason, I put excellence in nutrition at the head of the list in improving and maintaining optimal brain function.

America's memory is failing, not only because the baby boom dictated long ago that a greater percent of our population would start getting older all at once (although that demographic truth does play a role) but also because the quality of the food we eat, as a nation, has declined with our addiction to convenience and speed. Instead of enjoying wholesome meals made of fresh ingredients, far too many of our meals come wrapped in plastic, flash frozen, quick fried, or nuked, and tucked into foam and are eaten on the run. Regardless of what appears to be in the wrapper, virtually all convenience foods consist mainly of sugar, refined starches, and poor-quality fats and oils, with the occasional bit of protein thrown in. A steady diet of cereal, toaster pastries, pizza, fast-food burgers, chips, fries, and sodas doesn't begin to pro- vide the brain with the quality raw materials it needs to function properly, let alone at its peak. If this diet resembles yours, we need to talk.

CHRONIC STRESS

In this day and age, it seems that stress is something we simply must learn to live with. If so, it's quite important to our health that we try to protect ourselves from it to as great an extent as possible. Although we humans were designed by nature to cope with brief episodes of sudden stress—running for our lives from something trying to eat us, for example—our Stone Age body systems are ill-prepared to withstand the constant pressures of juggling work, home, bills, phone calls, church, kids, school, community activities, and the information overload we're exposed to day in and day out.

Research in laboratory animals has shown this type of chronic stress damages certain delicate parts of the brain associated with memory and learning. In people, persistently elevated levels of the stress hormone cortisol—even borderline high levels that are still technically within the normal range—have been shown to impair memory and to be associated with shrinkage of key memory areas of the brain, such as the fragile area known as the hippocampus. In the normal course of events, cortisol levels fall during sleep and rise during our waking hours, however, the levels tend to remain persistently elevated during periods of sleep deprivation.

Moreover, chronic stress can lead to mild depression or anxiety and interfere with our ability to sleep soundly. But we probably don't need lab research to prove to us that working long hours on little sleep isn't healthy for the body or the brain; most of us have been there and know it firsthand.

Because the brain consumes energy 10 times faster than the remainder of the body, a sound, healthy night's sleep—while the rest of the body is quiet and still and the power requirements are lower—leaves more energy production available to allow the brain to reenergize and catch up.

SLEEP DEPRIVATION

The body needs rest, but the brain needs sleep. The miracle of sleep is what allowed our amazing brains to evolve to their present configuration; it's what preserves their ongoing healthy function. And yet, according to a recent study by the National Sleep Foundation, one in five Americans routinely suffers from lack of sleep. That's 20 percent of us, tired, confused, and unable to properly (let alone optimally) perform tasks that require sharp, focused thinking, or quick reaction.

Some of us lack sufficient sleep because of work. The all-nighters pulled by college and med students cramming for exams and by doctors, nurses, police officers, firefighters, military personnel, long-haul truckers, and shift workers—and, nowadays, even lawyers, accountants, and MBAs in the routine course of their careers—have become so common as to be an expected requirement of these jobs. Putting in 14-, 18-, even 20-hour workdays; pulling double shifts; working weekends; and skipping vacations may get you ahead of the financial curve, but it leaves precious little time for sleep. And ultimately, the lack will take its toll. Studies have demonstrated that going without sleep for 20 hours impairs reactions as much as alcohol levels considered illegal in most states.

But long hours aren't the only reason for sleep deprivation. Even those lucky enough to make it to bed at a reasonable hour and stay there for the recommended 8 hours may not sleep well. We toss, turn, awaken with gastric reflux or heartburn and stress over money, work, kids, and other issues, all of which interferes with getting a restful night's sleep. Some of us (particularly those with diabesity) may develop a dangerous and potentially fatal disorder called sleep apnea, in which breathing stops for short periods of time throughout the night, prompting loud snoring, thrashing about, poor-quality sleep, and fatigue and sleepiness the following day. Remember, the body needs rest, but the brain needs sleep. Sound, natural sleep.

Natural sleep progresses in cycles, as throughout the night we drift into and out of several stages that differ mainly in the speed of the brain waves generated during them and the presence or absence of muscle activity. From the fast transmission that occurs when we're awake, the brain waves become progressively slower as we fall more and more deeply asleep. Periodically in these prolonged stretches of slow waves, the sleeping brain enters special cycles called rapid eye movement (REM) sleep, a phenomenon that, it is interesting to note, occurs only in warm-blooded animals. Scientists now believe that, in humans at least, the phases of natural sleep serve, to put it in computer terms, as offline processing time to allow the brain to deal with the enormous amount of sensory (especially visual) information we receive each day. Furthermore, research indicates that adequate amounts of both these types of sleep are critical to the consolidation and reinforcement of memories and learning.

Interesting studies done in young healthy male volunteers have shown that even a few days of sleep loss (on average sleeping about 4 hours a night) can disturb the metabolic systems that regulate blood sugar. This produces transient glucose intolerance to the degree seen in diabetes. When these young subjects resumed sleeping for 9 hours each night, the metabolic changes resolved. And that's good news.

Chronic sleep deprivation, no matter what the cause, stresses the brain and interferes with the normal nightly drop in stress hormones, such as cortisol, which then build up to higher than normal levels. Persistent elevation of this hormone over a several month period has been shown by MRI scans of the brain to actually shrink the hippocampus, the region responsible for accurate memory. Moreover, chronically high cortisol levels not only produce insulin resistance and elevate blood sugar (both major risks for memory loss) but also impair the ability of brain cells to generate energy, disrupt their calcium metabolism, and even make them more vulnerable to the physical or toxic insults of the environment.

Fortunately, by restoring a pattern of sound, natural sleep and thereby lowering the level of cortisol, the hippocampus can usually recover. MRI scans of the brain have actually documented the recovery of a previously shriveled hippocampus by restoring sleep. If lack of sleep is leaving you in a mental fog and robbing you of memory, restoring natural sleep is of paramount importance to your brain health. This program will provide the proper nutritional framework, and helpful tips and tricks will let you sleep soundly once again.

BEATING YOUR HEAD AGAINST A WALL

Head injury is one of the fairly self-evident environmental risk factors that can rob us of memory and mental sharpness. We all know of, or at least have seen on television, someone who's been knocked out by a fist, a fall, or a football helmet. We've witnessed the dazed expressions on their faces, the blank stares from their eyes, and their visible confusion in not knowing what ZIP code they're in, much less recalling what just happened. Concussions, even mild ones with brief loss of consciousness, clearly disrupt short-term memory, often resulting in transient amnesia, difficulty recalling words or faces, and slowed reaction speed. The fuzzy head from such an injury can last minutes to weeks to, in some cases, a lifetime. A blow to the head, associated with loss of consciousness for an hour or more, can double the risk of developing memory deficits (even Alzheimer's disease) later in life.

President Reagan, for instance, suffered a blow to his head related to a fall from a horse not long before his physician team diagnosed Alzheimer's disease. Let me hasten to say that I do not intend to imply that the fall caused his disease; however, when the delicate areas of the brain involved in memory and learning begin to shrink and deteriorate and their function is marginal, a severe blow to the head can be the straw that breaks the camel's back by placing added stress on an already struggling organ.

In the wake of Reagan's devastating ordeal, scientific investigation has proceeded apace into the causes, nature, and course in Alzheimer's and related conditions. And some of that research has demonstrated evidence of a link between head injury and the subsequent development of chronic and progressive dementing illnesses (such as Alzheimer's disease) and the development of chronic and progressive degenerative illnesses of the brain and nervous system (such as Parkinson's disease).

Although you can't always guard against accidents—you may slip, you may fall, you may be struck in the head by an errant pitch—you wouldn't sign up for it voluntarily. After all, most of us don't bang our heads against a wall on purpose. Or do we? In a sense, it happens quite often in sports. In some cases, such as boxing, football, and soccer, the risk of being banged in the head is obvious. For others, such as jogging and Bungee jumping, it's much less apparent, because the damage is caused not from a singular blow to the head from without, but from repetitively banging the brain against the skull from within.

You see, the brain is such a delicate and critically important organ that nature has encased it in thick bony armor—the skull—in which it floats in a cushioning layer of protective fluid. But even this degree of protection isn't foolproof. Because the brain does float a bit, in a sport, such as Bungee jumping, the sudden jerk that stops the fall can snap the head and thump the brain against the bony inside of the skull. Fortunately, most people don't Bungee jump on a daily basis. However, in the same if less dramatic way, the chronic, repetitive pound, pound, pounding of jogging—an activity regularly engaged in by an estimated 30 million people in the United States and to an extreme degree by nearly 400,000 marathon runners—can cause the brain to thud, thud, thud within the fluid cushion inside the skull.

One fairly sensitive tool that scientists have developed to assess the degree of actual brain trauma from head injury is the measurement of a specific protein, released by the injured brain, called S-100B, which can be detected in blood. Studies have shown that patients whose blood tests high for the S-100B protein after a mild head injury have a higher likelihood of developing brain or memory deficits. Furthermore, the S-100B levels are higher in boxers, whose heads clearly take a beating. Research has even shown that some long-distance joggers have as much S-100B in their blood as boxers do. It is not known what this means for joggers' long-term brain health, but the connection is unsettling all the same. For people with other risk factors for memory loss, running could prove to be a counterproductive strategy, at least for brain health.

"Great," you may be thinking, "I'll just opt out of exercise, live the life of a couch potato, and save my brain!" Think again. Unfortunately, the other side of the exercise coin with regard to brain health is that it's not good to be sedentary either. In fact, research implicates a sedentary lifestyle as a risk for memory loss in its own right.

For brain health, the key is to remain active but to choose an activity that doesn't beat your head against the figurative wall. Regular, sensible exercise promotes the release of certain beneficial substances, such as brain-derived neurotrophic factor (BDNF). BNDF promotes brain growth, rebuilding, and repair. It behooves us to do what we can to make more BDNF available—that is, if building and maintaining a healthy, optimally functioning brain is our goal.

HARDENING OF THE ARTERIES AND HIGH BLOOD PRESSURE

A vast network of arteries ferries blood from the heart to every nook and cranny of the body from the tip of the nose to the ends of the toes, delivering the nutrients and oxygen our tissues need to survive and thrive. When we're young our blood vessels are supple and clean; but for some, if not most of us, time takes its toll. And, like the plumbing in an aging house, the vessels narrow with deposits and become stiffer. This hardening process—called arteriosclerosis—can occur in vessels anywhere, from the big aorta that sends blood from the heart to the entire body, to the tiny coronary arteries that feed the heart, to the carotid and vertebral arteries in the neck that supply the blood to the head and brain.

Stiffness and narrowing of blood vessels can elevate blood pressure. Why? Think of what happens to the pressure when you crimp the end of a water hose, if the flow of water stays the same: the water spews out at high pressure around the crimp. Smaller hole, higher pressure, it's a simple matter of physics.

About 25 percent of adults have elevated blood pressure, although only about one third of them know it. Because studies indicate that high blood pressure may be a major underlying cause of memory loss with age, it behooves us all to get it checked and, if it's elevated, take steps to bring it down.

But beyond just elevating pressure, arteriosclerosis within the system can have a variety of other consequences. For instance, narrowing of the blood vessels supplying the heart muscle can result in angina (heart pain) first with activity, then even at rest. If the flow is blocked entirely, a heart attack is the result. When deposits narrow the carotid or vertebral arteries, the reduced flow robs the brain of sufficient oxygen, glucose, and other critical nutrients. Like the oxygen-starved heart, a brain in need of oxygen can't function adequately, much less at its peak.

Moreover, small bits of the hardened plaques inside these arteries or blood clots that form around them can occasionally dislodge and travel downstream to plug narrower areas, blocking blood flow entirely to a portion of the brain, causing what's called an ischemic stroke. Another type of stroke, called a hemorrhagic stroke, can occur when elevated blood pressure blows out a weakened area in the diseased wall of an artery feeding the brain. In either event, the portions of the brain that rely on the disrupted blood supply will not fare well, and the affected brain cells will sicken and often die. Symptoms can range from numbness or tingling to disturbances in speech or memory to difficulty writing, speaking, or walking, depending on which areas of the brain the stroke involves.

Sometimes, however, the small bits of plaque or clot occlude the artery only momentarily, cutting off the supply of oxygen and nutrient-rich blood long enough to cause transient symptoms of numbness, vision change, loss of normal speech or movement that resolve within 24 hours or so. These transient ischemic attacks (TIAs)—or mini-strokes, as they're often called—may cause less immediate damage, but there is damage nevertheless. Repeated small attacks will finally take their toll on memory and brain function.

What causes arteries to harden? The current thinking is that low-level chronic inflammation lies at the root of plaque formation in the arteries, whether in the aorta, the coronary arteries, the carotids, the vertebrals, or the smaller vessels that feed the brain. Among the risk factors for its development, insulin resistance, diabetes, and hypertension seem to have starring roles; and certainly there's a genetic component. But perhaps the biggest player of all—and one we can choose to modify—is cigarette smoking. In fact, a recent study followed more than 1,000 people for 5 years in an attempt to correlate these risk factors with the development of Alzheimer's disease.

The researchers found that having three or more of them increased the risk of development of Alzheimer's disease by a whopping 340 percent, with smoking being one of the strongest predictors.

SMOKING

Because the universe of known risks associated with this behavior are many and varied, it should come as no surprise that smoking is hazardous to the memory. As is often the case, what's not good for the heart, lungs, skin, and body in general is also not good for the brain . . . only more so. One study, published in the scientific brain journal *Neurology* in 1999 showed that smoking doubles a person's risk for developing Alzheimer's disease. Based on that statistic, it would be reasonable to assume that smoking also increases the chance of developing less severe forms of memory loss. Why is smoking such a bad thing for the brain? The list is long and mostly toxic.

To begin with, the fumes of burning tobacco, like burning plastic or Teflon, are poisonous. Each puff of cigarette smoke contains not only the nicotine for which it is famous—or infamous—but carbon monoxide and about 4,000 other identified toxic compounds as well. While it's true that the body goes to great lengths to prevent toxins from passing out of the blood and into the brain, it's also true that the protective shield, called the blood–brain barrier, is not foolproof. Some substances do make it through. That's why humans can get high from sniffing glue, become drunk on alcohol, or catch a buzz from smoking a cigarette. Despite the blood–brain barrier, these substances pass from the lungs or stomach, into the blood, and on into the brain. And because the brain is made largely of delicate fats, many of these toxic compounds can dissolve in the fatty membranes and tissues, poison the brain cells, and damage or kill them. In addition, smoking has been implicated as one culprit in the development of other brain health risk factors, such as insulin resistance, hardening of the arteries, and high blood pressure.

The good news for smokers is that quitting, at any age, reduces the risk. Recent statistics estimate that 46 million adult Americans smoke and that about 70 percent of them say they'd like to quit. If you smoke, you're at greater risk for memory impairment and Alzheimer's disease. If you're worried about the sharpness of your memory, quitting smoking is an important first step to preserving and improving it. Take that step. Use patches, use gum, use nasal inhalers, use hypnosis—but by some means, if you care for your brain, stop smoking.

ALCOHOL USE

Alcohol's effect on the brain and on memory proves you can get too much of a good thing. As is the case with heart health and weight control, it appears with the brain that drinking a modest amount of alcohol—on the order of a single drink most days—is better for brain health than total abstinence. Results of studies designed to test the association between alcoholism and confirmed dementia indicate that people having 1 drink a week lower their risk of memory decline by 35 percent over teetotalers; those who imbibe 1 to 6 drinks a week reduce their risk by 54 percent. The protective effect begins to decline a bit to a 31 percent reduction in those who have 7 to 13 drinks a week, and the protection vanishes entirely thereafter. People who regularly drink 14 or more drinks a week have a 22 percent greater risk of developing dementia as they age.

Most of us are well acquainted with the short-term effect of too much alcohol on brain function. Blood levels as low as 0.02 percent can impair our ability to operate a car or machinery. Higher levels can make us unable to walk straight, to speak clearly, and may even render us unconscious. Chronic alcoholism not only results in various amnesia and blackout syndromes but has also been suspected as a cause of brain shrinkage.

Alcohol is a toxic substance. It is basically a fat solvent that the liver must detoxify and eliminate. From that perspective, it's easy to see why consuming a lot of it could harm the brain, which is mostly made of fat. What's not as clear is why a little of it would be beneficial to the brain. And in fact, exactly why a modest intake of alcohol would confer memory protection isn't yet clearly understood, although neuroscientists continue to try to unravel the underlying mechanism.

MEDICATIONS

Even the best drugs can have serious side effects. Some of them affect the brain, either by depleting critical nutrients or by directly impairing thinking and memory. The brain is made mostly of delicate fats that are particularly susceptible to oxidization—or in the vernacular, to going rancid. To prevent this, the body supplies the brain richly with antioxidants, particularly with the natural antioxidant compound coenzyme Q10 (CoQ_{10}). This critical protective nutrient not only acts to keep the brain's delicate fats fresh and functional but is also essential for the production of energy in the power-generating parts of the brain cells. An important role, because a cellular power shortage leads to sluggish brain function, slowed reaction times, fatigue, and loss of mental acuity.

One large and frequently prescribed class of drugs falls into the first category, that of depleting a critical nutrient. The statin drugs, commonly used for cholesterol lowering, deplete one of the brain's critical antioxidant protectors. This class of drugs works to lower cholesterol by interfering with the action of a particular enzyme that controls the production of cholesterol in the liver. Unfortunately, this enzyme also controls the production of CoQ_{10}. Taking a statin, whether Lipitor, Crestor, Zocor, Mevacor, Pravachol, or some other, may cut your CoQ_{10} levels in half and put your memory at risk. And the potential for nerve cell damage doesn't stop at the head; people taking these medications also sometimes report numbness and tingling in the extremities; in fact, they do so 16 times more often than those who do not take them.

But statins aren't the only class of drugs that can deplete CoQ_{10}. Other commonly prescribed drugs that can do so include major antidepressant and tranquilizing medications (Elavil, Sinequan, Tofranil, Haldol), blood pressure medications (Tenormin, Catapres, Dyazide, Toprol, Inderal), and diabetes medications (Glucotrol, Micronase, Tolinase.) If you must take one of these medications, for the sake of your brain you should also supplement your diet with extra CoQ_{10} each day.

Another group of critical brain nutrients often interfered with or depleted by commonly prescribed medications is the family of B vitamins, low levels of which have been implicated for centuries in symptoms ranging from mood disorders and memory loss to frank dementia. In the post–civil war South, mental asylums were filled with people thought to be insane, who were merely suffering from the vitamin deficiency disorder known as pellagra from subsisting on B vitamin–depleted cornmeal as their staple. More recently, research has uncovered another mechanism through which deficiency of the B family members folic acid, B_6 and B_{12} may affect brain function. We now know that these vitamins play a crucial role in the proper handling of a substance called homocysteine, a normal byproduct generated by certain body processes. Homocysteine is quite toxic if not inactivated or recycled properly—a job requiring an adequate supply of these B vitamins. When elevated, it increases the risk for stroke, heart attack, and even Alzheimer's disease.

A wide array of common medications can interfere with B vitamin levels: aspirin, diuretics (fluid or water pills) used for high blood pressure, stomach acid blockers (such as Nexium and Prilosec), estrogen-containing birth control and hormone-replacement pills (such as Ortho-Novum, Ortho-TriCyclen, Premarin, Prempro, and CombiPatch), drugs used to combat osteoporosis (such as Fosamax, Actonel, and Evista), and the most widely prescribed drug for the treatment for Parkinson's disease (Sinemet). With the exception of birth control pills, these are drugs primarily prescribed to older people; the group who can least withstand added insult to the brain. Depletion of B vitamins and the consequent rise in homocysteine it causes present a double whammy to the aging brain.

Other medications can directly disrupt mental function, causing drowsiness, slowing thought processes and reaction speed, and causing foggy thinking. Almost any medication that comes with a warning that it should not be taken with alcoholic beverages will fall into this group. Drugs designed to cause sedation or relaxation are the obvious candidates, including such medications as tranquilizers, sleeping pills, medications to combat depression or anxiety, muscle relaxants, and seizure medications. When taken as directed, the effects on the brain are usually mild and temporary. Stopping the medication usually resolves the symptoms without lasting effect.

I've said, there are two basic ways that medications can have an effect on brain function, but a final group—the potent anti-inflammatory agents called corticosteroids, or simply steroids[2]—can actually damage brain health in a third way, by mimicking the unwanted effect of a natural substance in the body. The use of steroid medications, such as those typified by the drug cortisone, can put the brain at risk in much the same way that chronic elevation of their natural counterpart, cortisol, does. Physicians usually prescribe these steroid medications for chronic disorders, such as severe allergies or asthma, Crohn's disease, ulcerative colitis, rheumatoid arthritis, SLE, and other similar major inflammatory or autoimmune diseases. Steroids have been called "wonder drugs," and indeed they are quite effective in treating these conditions, which often fail to respond to other therapies. For some people, it may be impossible to completely avoid their use; however, most doctors will agree that it's important to use them sparingly and to limit their use to the shortest possible time to get the job done. As is the case with too much natural cortisol, prolonged use of steroids impairs the ability of brain and nerve cells to resist insults, making them more prone to lose their connections to other cells.

ILLICIT DRUGS

Remember the long-running television ad campaign from Partnership for a Drug-Free America back in the 1980s and 1990s? "This is your brain. This is your brain on drugs." One of these ads showed a raw egg being dropped onto a very hot skillet to illustrate the point that drugs can fry your brain. This message packed a wallop and got the point across. Commonly used street drugs clearly damage the brain and, unfortunately, too often with lasting impact. Let's look briefly at what the four most commonly abused illicit drugs can do to a brain.

Amphetamine, termed speed in the vernacular, and its derivatives top the list of abused drugs that adversely affect the brain, primarily because their abuse is so widespread. These stimulant compounds send the blood pressure

2. These are not the illegal steroids abused by some athletes, which include male sex hormones or their precursors.

into the stratosphere, often sufficiently to cause a stroke, even in young brains. It should come as no surprise that hemorrhage into the brain isn't good for it, but that's not the only way this group of drugs can cause damage. Recent research has shown that speed causes actual changes in the brain cells, leaving protein deposits strikingly similar to those seen in the brains of people with degenerative brain disorders, such as Alzheimer's disease.

Research from the University of Michigan suggests that cocaine can actually destroy certain cells in the brain that produce the natural feel-good chemical messenger called dopamine. In fact, the high that people get from using cocaine comes about because the drug causes a surge in the brain's production of dopamine, leading to a sense of euphoria. Chronic use of cocaine—which all too often follows casual use—can deplete and finally destroy the cells that make dopamine, leaving the brain deprived of this important regulatory chemical and the brain's owner at heightened risk for developing Parkinson's disease. If that weren't enough, cocaine's stimulating properties can also raise blood pressure sufficiently to increase the risk for stroke.

Developed originally in Germany as an appetite suppressant, ecstasy (MDMA) took the nation's nightclub scene by storm not only for its stimulant effects, which allow users to dance all night long at raves or techno parties, but also for its hallucinogenic effect that users claim heightens their senses and removes their inhibitions. The drug actually enters the brain where it produces the high by causing a sudden excess of serotonin to develop. With continued use, this action paradoxically produces depletion of this important chemical, the loss of which can be deadly for the cell. The hallucinogenic effects most likely occur when the surge of serotonin acts on certain of its receptors, called the psychedelic receptors. These brain receptors are also affected by the classic hallucinogenic drugs LSD, psilocybin, and mescaline. The stimulating effects are associated with elevated heart rate, blood pressure, and risk for stroke.

Studies have documented memory loss associated with ecstasy use; the $64,000 question is, Are the losses temporary or permanent? To answer that question, a recent study compared people still using the drug with people who had stopped. Those who continued to use the drug, logically enough, appeared to suffer continued memory decline. It is interesting, however, that the memories of some of the now-abstinent users remained impaired; but the memories of others slightly improved, suggesting that at least in some people ecstasy's effect on memory might be reversible. Good news indeed.

After its heyday in the 1960s and 1970s, marijuana has made a comeback in the last decade and is once again the most commonly abused illicit drug in the United States. Although thought by some to be a relatively harmless intoxicant, the mind-altering effects of pot smoking in the short term can include problems with memory and learning, distorted perceptions, difficulty with thinking and problem solving, and loss of coordination. The effect on the brain of its long-term use remains somewhat unclear; however, a recent study points to lasting effects from prolonged use.

Researchers compared the performance of 20 long-term pot users, 20 short-term users, and 24 non-user controls on various tests of memory, ability to focus, and mental agility or quickness. Long-term users scored significantly worse on verbal memory and on mental quickness than either short-term users or controls. Both long-term and short-term users demonstrated deficits in verbal fluency, verbal memory, attention, and mental quickness compared to the non-users. The investigators concluded that particular areas of brain function involving memory deteriorate with prolonged heavy use.

Warning Signs: Loss of Hearing and Loss of Smell

For the brain to make sense of our surroundings it must sample the environment; it does so by sending what amount to data gathering probes to the surface. We know these probes as sensory organs—our eyes, ears, nose, tongue, and skin. The nerve endings that allow us to see, hear, smell, taste, and feel connect directly to brain cells. In effect, these sensory organs are merely extensions of the brain and, as such, can serve as clues to the brain's health. Two of our senses in particular—smell and hearing—can act as bellwethers of brain health. You'll find more information about this topic in Chapter 7, but for now, be aware that people who experience dulling of these two senses may be at heightened risk for memory decline and even Alzheimer's disease with age.

People can usually perceive that their sense of hearing isn't what it used to be, or at least their spouse or family members can. Getting your hearing checked by an audiologist is a fairly simple matter. The good news is that you can protect your hearing from further loss through better nutrition; in subsequent chapters you'll learn how.

Loss of sense of smell is a little trickier and may slip by unnoticed for quite some time. You'll find a 10-item smell test in Chapter 7 that will help you determine if you've lost some of your ability to identify odors that could point to a need for further investigation by your physician to determine the cause.

Now that you know where you fall on the spectrum of risk and you're better acquainted with how the various risk factors affect brain health, it's time to take a look at what you can do about it. My Brain Trust Program will positively influence the health and performance of your brain. It can help you prevent further loss, strengthen your memory, improve your focus, lift the mental fog, and ensure that your brain functions at its peak for the long haul.

The take home message from this chapter on risk factors is to realize that with the exception of family history, you can do something about virtually every single one. Subsequent chapters show you exactly how to do it.

PART II

The Three-Part Brain Trust Program

4

The Care and Feeding of the Brain: What (and What Not) to Eat

There's very little value in discovering that you're at risk for something if there's nothing you can do about it but worry. Not so very long ago scientific dogma suggested that the brain was a wasting asset and that with the passage of each day, we lost many millions of brain cells that could not be replaced. Experts once believed we were born with a given number of brain cells, and that was that. With age, memory would fail us and some of us would see our mental faculties gradually fade into senility. A bleak picture if I ever saw one.

Fortunately for us all, and contrary to the perceived wisdom of those days, we now understand that there's a lot we can do to preserve, protect, and even improve brain function from *birth to old age*. Science has proven that instead of being static, the brain not only can but indeed actually does form millions of new synapses (the interconnections that allow brain cells to communicate) every day of our lives, no matter what our age. Better still, researchers at several laboratories have documented that brand-new, functional nerve cells can form in mature adult brains and not just a few, but legions of them, 25,000 or more a day. To make that happen, you've got to properly feed and care for your brain, starting now. Let's see how.

Many of the factors that come together to rob us of memory as we age involve specific lifestyle choices, completely within our control and, therefore, are risks we can do something about if we choose to. It's a concept very much like changing the way we eat or live to reduce our risk of heart disease. Just as we can rehabilitate a frail or failing body or heart through the right diet, nutritional supplements, and exercise, we can breathe new life into an aging brain or even one damaged by stroke or trauma using the same basic ideas. With the brain, it's just a bit trickier to do. And here's why.

When you eat food or take a nutritional supplement, you can assume that whatever it is you've eaten or taken will be absorbed into your bloodstream and reliably make its way to your heart, muscles, internal organs, or bones to nourish them. Not so with the brain. Because it's mostly made of fat, the brain is exceptionally susceptible to toxic damage. Any substance that can dissolve in oil—a long list that includes many pesticides, herbicides, hormones, growth factors, pollutants, and medications—could easily cross from the blood into the brain, where it could wreck havoc on the delicate fats that make up the lion's share of the brain's substance. To forestall such an occurrence, nature has designed the brain with several virtually fail-safe protections, among them a filtering system called the blood–brain barrier. This filter screens the blood as it goes by and allows only approved substances to pass through the barrier to get into the brain. I use the term *virtually* because, like Achilles, the seemingly invincible warrior of Homer's *Iliad*, the brain has one tiny chink in its armor, one small spot left unprotected, called the bare area of the blood–brain barrier. Through this small rent in the barrier, some substances can sneak across, and not all of them are good. You can think of the bare area as the Achilles' heel of the brain.

In some ways, the blood–brain barrier functions too well. As is often the case, a system designed to protect us from harm can also serve to limit our access to that which might do us good. Consequently, if any supplement or medication is to get into the brain to nourish or heal, it must be in a form that can cross this barrier. This fact comes into play in selecting which foods we should eat and which forms of supplements we should take to optimize brain function. I'll delve more deeply into supplementation in a later chapter, but first let's look at what constitutes a brain-friendly diet.

The Brain-Friendly Diet: What to Eat

For general good health, I think everyone can agree that we should eat a widely varied, nutritious diet. Granted, not everyone agrees on exactly what that means; is it low carb, low fat, low calorie, high protein? As a general dictum, "Eat a varied, nutritious diet" won't ruffle the feathers of proponents of virtually any of the main nutritional camps. For the purposes of benefiting the brain and optimizing brain function, however, there are some foods that stand out as being of special importance. Among them are fish and seafood, berries, spinach, certain herbs and spices, green tea, coffee, eggs, avocado, nuts, seeds, and wine. Let me hasten to say that these are not the only foods I recommend that you eat. (I'll outline some meal plans for the Brain Trust Program a little later.) They are simply the foods that I think—and science has shown—offer the most direct benefit to the brain. Here's why I feel each of these plays an important role in any brain healthy diet.

Essential fatty acids fall into one of two categories—omega-3s or omega-6s. Because the brain contains the highest concentration of long-chain omega-3 fatty acids in the body, and because they are primarily found in fish and seafood, these foods find themselves at the top of the list. Located in the outer coating of the nerve cells where the neurotransmitter molecules bind and enable cellular communication, these fats are critical in every function the brain undertakes.

Because they are so sensitive to oxidation, or going rancid, these delicate fats need to be protected by an array of natural compounds called antioxidants. These are abundant in fruits, vegetables, and spices, which is why berries, spinach, coffee, and avocados are so vital for brain health. Eggs, nuts, and seeds are good sources of multiple brain healthy nutrients, including monounsaturated fats, vitamins, and minerals. Last, but not least, wine, in moderation has been shown to be an excellent source of resveratrol and many powerful flavonoid antioxidants.

FISH AND SEAFOOD

When I was a child I was taught that fish is brain food; you probably were, too. It turns out that the old wives' tale we learned as kids is right on the money, as a team of researchers in the Chicago Health and Aging Project recently proved. The research team examined the diet histories of and performed brain-specific tests on more than 4,000 people. These people were then followed for 6 years. The team found that those who ate the most fish had better preserved memory functions than those who ate little or no fish. Or, put a different way, the study showed that eating fish significantly slowed the decline in mental function that occurs with age.

What is it about fish that is so good for the brain? Certainly, fish are a good source of top-quality protein, important not just for building the brain but for building a healthy body as well. More important for the brain, however, is that fish—particularly those that thrive in the deep cold waters of the ocean or in snow-fed mountain streams (salmon, mackerel, tuna, sardines, and trout)—are a rich source of the essential fats that the brain depends on to work properly.

These special fats, called omega-3 fatty acids, are highly unsaturated molecules that give the cell membranes throughout the body—including the brain cells—the flexibility and fluidity necessary to function properly. More on this topic later.

It's actually the algae living in the cold waters that produce the critical omega-3 fatty acids; the fish come by them secondhand. When the fish eat the algae, the omega-3s get tucked away in their fat cells or in their livers. Fish that live in cold water contain more fat and can, therefore, store more omega-3 fatty acids, which is why they are our best nutritional source for this important class of brain nutrients. Unfortunately, the fat of fish, like the fat that makes up our brains, is also a good place to store heavy metals, pesticides, polychlorinated biphenyls (PCBs), and other toxic chemicals, which add a layer of complexity to the equation. I'll go into this topic in more detail later, but suffice it to say now that in general smaller fish (sardines) will be freer of toxins than larger fish (tuna).

In the brain, these essential fats play several important roles. First, and possibly most important, the brain cells weave them into the structure of their cell membranes to keep them pliable and help them work properly. Embedded within the membrane of every brain cell are special structures, called receptors, which serve as activation switches for critical brain activities. If the membranes become too stiff, key brain chemicals can't trigger these activation switches. When this occurs, critical brain activities such as learning, reaction speed, and memory begin to decline.

Good fish sources of omega-3s are salmon, tuna, mackerel, herring, trout, sardines, and anchovies. And remember that, generally speaking, the smaller the fish, the fewer the toxins. Table 4.1 provides a list of the omega-3 fatty acid content of common food fish.

BERRIES

Eating a variety of fresh fruits and vegetables is important for overall good health and brain health is no exception. Science has identified thousands of plant-based chemicals that seem to have benefit in human health, many of them associated with the pigments that give the fruit or vegetable its color. And while it might be nice to isolate them into a simple pill or two, the rub is that they seem to work best in concert in ways that, as yet, science can't mimic. Science can, however, measure their function and doing so yields a value, called the oxygen radical absorbance capacity (ORAC), that quantifies the ability of any food substance to neutralize oxygen free-radicals.

Although prunes and raisins are highest of all, of the fresh fruits, berries top the ORAC charts; they are nutrient dense but contain less concentrated sugars than their dried-fruit cousins. For this reason, berries are an especially important high-ORAC foods source in a brain healthy diet for people with obesity, diabetes, or other insulin-resistance related disease, in whom control of excess sugar assumes even greater importance.

TABLE 4.1

Amount of Omega-3 Fatty Acids in Fish and Seafood*

FISH/SEAFOOD	OMEGA-3 (GRAMS PER 3-OUNCE SERVING)
Tuna	
Light, canned in water	0.26
White, canned in water	0.73
Fresh	0.24–1.28
Sardine	0.98–1.70
Salmon	
Sockeye	0.68
Pink	1.09
Chinook	1.48
Atlantic, farmed	1.09–1.83
Atlantic, wild	0.9–1.56
Mackerel	0.34–1.57
Herring	
Pacific	1.81
Atlantic	1.71
Trout, rainbow	
Farmed	0.98
Wild	0.84
Halibut	0.4–1.0
Cod	
Atlantic	0.24
Pacific	0.13
Haddock	0.2
Flounder	0.42
Oyster	
Pacific	1.17
Eastern	0.47
Farmed	0.37
Lobster	0.07–0.41
Crab, Alaskan King	0.35
Shrimp	0.27
Clam	0.24
Scallop	0.17

*Data from H. Iso, M. Kobayashi, J. Ishihara, S. Sasaki, K. Okada, Y. Kita, Y. Kokubo, and S. Tsugane. "Intake of Fish and ω3 Fatty Acids and Risk of Coronary Heart Disease among Japanese." *Circulation* 113 (2006): 195–202.

The delicate fats that make up so great a part of the brain's structure—the very ones I encourage you to replace by eating cold-water fish—are quite vulnerable to attack by oxygen, which is, of course, a necessary part of life. Eating foods with a high ORAC content not only helps protect essential brain fats from oxidation but can also protect the skin, heart, and eyes. Research suggests that simply eating more of these foods may also help prevent memory loss and improve learning ability. Since they're delicious, it's a pretty easy assignment.

SPINACH AND OTHER DARK GREEN LEAFY VEGETABLES

While we've known it for many years as the strength builder that made Popeye "strong to the finish," the brain building powers of spinach have only recently come to light. Spinach, like the colorful fruits, is an ORAC superstar, which means, of course, that it has the antioxidant power to whip oxygen free-radicals like Popeye whipped Bluto. Filled with an array of antioxidant and anti-inflammatory compounds that research has shown will slow brain aging, improve memory, and enhance dexterity, spinach is one of the few food sources of the versatile antioxidant, α-lipoic acid (I'll delve much more deeply into the importance of this particular antioxidant to the brain in the next chapter.)

Spinach is also rich in the B vitamin folic acid, one of the chief weapons deployed by the body to neutralize homocysteine, an amino acid byproduct of the breakdown of another important amino acid called methionine. The primary food sources of methionine—an essential amino acid for humans, meaning we must eat it to live—are meat, fish, and poultry; but it's also found in tofu, fruits, nuts, kidney and black turtle beans, peas, corn, some cheeses, garlic, and—oddly enough—spinach. Most of us are able to take the homocysteine we produce naturally from the methionine we must eat and, using folic acid, turn it back into methionine. Some people, however, inherit a genetic difficulty in handling homocysteine, and the amino acid builds up in their bloodstreams, where it promotes atherosclerosis (hardening of the arteries) and predisposes them to heart attack, stroke, bone thinning, and dementia.

According to the Framingham Study data, high homocysteine levels can increase the risk for Alzheimer's disease in people over age 60 by as much as 150 percent.

But homocysteine levels can also rise in people who do not inherit the homocysteine metabolism disorder. Research shows that people with diabetes and those with insulin resistance disorder—both of which, as you will see throughout this book, put the brain at increased risk for memory failure with age—have a heightened risk for elevated homocysteine and a tougher time keeping its level near normal. In addition, the high levels of homocysteine exert a much more powerful effect on the health of people with diabetes than those without the disorder.

I encourage you to consume spinach and its dark green leafy relatives (turnip, mustard, and collard greens; kale; and chard) regularly. Eat them fresh in salads, sauté them in olive oil, or toss them into soups or stews.

SPICES

Prized by virtually every cuisine in the world, spices have been used for millennia to enhance the flavor or color of food and even to heal illness. The quest for spices sparked wars, built fortunes, floated entire economies, and resulted in the European discovery of the Americas. A secret blend of 11 herbs and spices even launched a fried-chicken empire. What are herbs and spices and why should they figure into a brain healthy plan of eating?

Although most people think of herbs and spices as being the same types of substances, there are differences between them. Herbs usually come from the green leafy parts of nonwoody plants, which we can use either fresh or dried to add flavor and vibrant color to food. The herbs thyme, rosemary, oregano, basil, chives, onion, garlic, cilantro, parsley, fennel, and dill are common to most household kitchens. Spices, on the other hand, are generally the whole or ground dried seeds, berries, bark, or roots of plants. Most of us are familiar with the spices cinnamon, cardamom, anise, coriander seed, mustard seed, hot chile, paprika, and black pepper. The distinction isn't really important for our purposes. Because we use small amounts of herbs and spices to provide flavor and color, rather than substance, to our foods, they offer an easy way to boost the intake of healthful nutrients in our diets without adding a lot of calories. Let's look at a few of these flavorings that science has shown to be beneficial to the brain, especially those that improve memory or prevent its loss with age.

Turmeric, a cousin of ginger, is the spice that gives Indian curries their bright yellow tint. This spice first attracted the attention of scientists researching Alzheimer's disease because rates of the disease are relatively low in India, where curry is a dietary staple. Scientific analysis has shown that one of the active ingredients in turmeric, a substance called curcumin, may prevent mental decline in laboratory animals. Lab research has also shown curcumin and *ginger* to sharply decrease the formation of the sticky deposits in the brain that are the hallmark of Alzheimer's disease. In addition, both ginger and curcumin suppress inflammation, which plays a major role in brain aging and disease.

A mountain of research has shown that *cinnamon*, a staple spice in holiday cooking and a perennial favorite flavor of kids and adults alike reduces inflammation and even has antioxidant power. Better still, it's been shown to help control blood sugar and improve insulin sensitivity; when these two improve, brain health follows.

The herbs *sage* and *rosemary* have been shown to be beneficial to brain health. The active ingredient in sage (the main herb of poultry seasoning) has been shown to boost the levels of acetylcholine, one of the chemicals responsible for transmitting messages within the memory centers of the brain. Some studies have shown that subjects who took sage oil improved short-term memory and the ability to recall words. Other research suggests that a substance in rosemary not only helps improve memory but also actually helps the brain to grow and repair the network of interconnections through which brain cells communicate with one another.

The plant chemicals that give an herb or spice its distinct flavor, strong aroma, and bright color often also account for its healthful properties. Adding a broad selection of healthful herbs and spices to the foods we eat is an easy and delicious way to benefit not only our brains but our overall health.

COFFEE

Researchers have repeatedly found that people who drink a couple of cups of caffeinated coffee each day have a lower incidence of Alzheimer's disease. Coffee—even decaf—contains several thousand antioxidant compounds, which may help keep us mentally sharp and slow brain decline with aging. Coffee drinking has also recently been shown to reduce the risk for developing diabetes, which is itself a powerful threat to memory.

Fortunately for noncoffee drinkers, research has also verified the same protection from drinking green tea. One study reported in the prestigious *American Journal of Clinical Nutrition* showed that drinking just one cup of green tea per day decreased the risk of declining mental abilities by 38 percent. Drinking a second one reduced the risk by 54 percent. The beneficial effects of drinking green tea may in part help explain the lower risk of memory decline and Alzheimer's disease in Japan, where green tea is a favored beverage. So enjoy at least a couple of daily cups of coffee or green tea; your brain will thank you.

EGGS

Make the versatile egg a regular part of your diet—all of it, including the yolk! And no, that is not a misprint. But before you gasp and say, "Eggs? Are you nuts? They're full of cholesterol; I can't eat eggs!" hear me out. Granted, in the last 15 years or so, the poor egg has been demonized (unfairly) as a health risk because of its cholesterol content; but, fortunately, science marches on and, as Bob Dylan once reminded us, the times, they are a'changin'.

While it's quite true that eggs are a source of cholesterol, science now agrees that eating them doesn't particularly raise the cholesterol level in your blood. In fact, dietary cholesterol only accounts for 10 to 15 percent of the cholesterol in your bloodstream. Your body, itself, makes the other 85 to

90 percent. In a fail-safe maneuver to be sure you have enough of this important raw material, if you eat less, your liver will simply crank up production.

What's more, you need cholesterol to make many hormones as well as vitamin D. It also plays a vital role as a structural molecule in the membrane of every cell in your body. The brain, especially, is a cholesterol-dependent organ. Research in animals, including nonhuman primates and humans, shows that deficiency of dietary cholesterol results in depression, aggression, and agitation. It is interesting that the average cholesterol level among prison inmates is lower than the average of the general population.

But eggs contain more than just cholesterol; they are an excellent and inexpensive source of complete protein and of important vitamins, such as A, E, B_{12}, and folate. The yolk is rich in lutein and zeaxanthin—two nutrients that research has shown will reduce the risk of macular degeneration of the eye. The macula is the most important portion of the retina, the screen at the back of the eye onto which we focus images to see. Macular degeneration is a leading cause of blindness. Also, don't forget that the eye is merely an extension of the brain, so it stands to reason that what's good for the eyes is good for the brain as a whole. But there's even more. Eggs are also rich in choline, another B vitamin family member and key player in maintaining brain health. Choline and folate work hand in hand to lower levels of homocysteine, which, if you recall, puts the brain at heightened risk for memory failure when allowed to build up. If you've been avoiding eggs because you thought they were bad for you, think again. If optimal brain health is your goal, it's time to bring the versatile egg back into your kitchen, yolk and all. As part of a sensible eating plan, it won't raise your cholesterol and your brain will thank you.

AVOCADOS

Eat more avocados, possibly the most nutritionally valuable fruit nature has given to us. Fruit? Surprising but true, the avocado is not a vegetable, but rather an oil-rich berry, like the olive, albeit a bit larger. And the oils it contains, mostly monounsaturated fats, help to keep the membranes of your brain cells (actually all your cells) appropriately flexible, so that they work optimally.

But good oils are only a part of the story; for instance, it may surprise you to learn that avocados contain more protein than cow's milk. Avocados are also bursting with other important nutrients, such as vitamins A, C, E, and K; the B complex vitamins; and folic acid—practically the whole alphabet of vitamins packed into one luscious fruit. Not only that, they're also rich in magnesium and potassium, two minerals crucial to optimal brain function and for which most Americans don't even come close to meeting the minimum daily recommended intake.

It's difficult to overstate the importance of magnesium in the human body because it's a key player in more than 300 chemical reactions, some of which include energy production, the conduction of nerve signals, and communication among cells. Magnesium, in particular, helps protect the brain cells from overstimulation, which can prove deadly to the cell. It accomplishes this nifty feat by blocking the entry of excess calcium into the cell's interior. You have learned about this topic of brain cell overstimulation, also called excitotoxicity, in Chapter 2. Suffice it to say at this point that magnesium is your best natural weapon against brain cell overstimulation, and any food rich in magnesium is one that you should eat regularly. Magnesium is notoriously hard to come by in food. However, dark green leafy vegetables, avocados, dairy products, and a few natural mineral waters contain moderate amounts of magnesium.

NUTS AND SEEDS

Nuts and seeds also contain a fair amount of magnesium and provide a tasty and highly portable way to get more magnesium into your diet along with good fats and oils. Seeds and nuts (which are actually also seeds, mainly of trees, just covered with a hard shell) of various types also provide other important nutrients for the brain. Plants go to great effort to produce seeds, filling them with high concentrations of vitamins, minerals, protein, and essential oils to give them the best possible chance of sprouting and carrying on the line. Incredibly, if stored carefully, some seeds can still sprout after 200 years. Although all nuts and seeds have good nutritional value, four stand out in my mind: flax, sunflower, sesame, and pumpkin. Let's take a look at them.

Flaxseeds are filled with healthy oils, almost 30 percent by weight; in particular, they are rich in α-linolenic acid (ALA), an omega-3 fatty acid that a healthy body can turn into the essential brain fats docosahexanoic acid (DHA) and eicosapentanoic acid (EPA). The rest of the seed is mainly fiber and protein along with a fair amount of vitamin E and carotene, which most seeds and nuts contain to help keep their rich store of fats fresh. The oil in flaxseeds is quite delicate and can easily become rancid, despite the natural antioxidants it contains, unless kept protected from air, heat, and light. Store both the seeds and the oil in airtight containers in the refrigerator for optimal freshness and do not heat the oil or use in cooking.

Sunflower seeds, the perennial favorite of backyard birds and baseball teams, are packed with protein and good oils; in fact, they're nearly half oil. But there's still room in those tiny little packets for a whole lot more: potassium, magnesium, phosphorus, and B vitamins to help generate brain cell energy and to curb the buildup of toxic homocysteine that can put memory at risk.

Sesame seeds, with more protein than eggs (gram per gram), were possibly humanity's first convenience food. They are portable, light, and easy to pack for long-distance travel. They're also an excellent source of minerals, B vitamins, and (with their husks on) one of the plant kingdom's best sources of calcium. Sesame seeds figure prominently into Asian, Indian, and Middle Eastern cooking, sprinkled on salads or in sautéed veggie and meat dishes. Try adding ground-up seeds or sesame seed butter, called *tahini*, to sauces or protein shakes.

Pumpkin seeds are another good source of protein, vitamins, and good fats. The seeds themselves, raw or roasted, make a great snack, but the oil is also quite tasty. Dark green with a full-bodied, buttery flavor, pumpkin seed oil provides another good source of beneficial omega-3 fatty acids, vitamin A, and calcium. It is a delicious alternative to olive oil for salad dressings.

WINE

Last, but certainly not least, I recommend enjoying a little wine, if you tolerate it. Many studies have shown that both men and women who drink a light to moderate amount—no more than one or two glasses a day—of wine, particularly red wine, suffer less memory decline and Alzheimer's disease than people who don't drink at all. It is interesting that beer doesn't provide this beneficial effect, so it's clearly not simply a matter of the alcohol in the wine, which research has shown raises high-density lipoprotein cholesterol (HDL), the good cholesterol. In fact, some studies show that those people who drink a light to moderate amount of beer may actually increase their risk for memory decline more than those who abstain from drinking.

So what is it in wine that's so beneficial to the brain? Some studies suggest that a natural substance found in wine called resveratrol may be responsible. A potent antioxidant and scavenger of free-radicals, resveratrol occurs mainly in the skins of red grapes, which leaches out into the grape juice as it sits on the skins during the fermentation process. Although both red and white wines are made from red grapes, the white wines aren't left to sit in the skins long enough to pick up the vibrant color; as a result the whites contain much less resveratrol than the reds and unfermented grape juice contains almost none. Moreover, the compound, being fat soluble, is absorbed far more readily in the presence of alcohol, its own natural solvent.

For those who can't tolerate alcohol, resveratrol is available in supplemental capsules. For those who can imbibe, enjoying a glass of red wine with dinner is good for the heart, good for the brain, and—if you like wine—just plain good!

The Brain-Friendly Diet: What *Not* to Eat

From before birth and throughout life, it's important to provide the brain with the raw materials it needs for growth and repair and to protect it from anything that might interfere with its optimal function. Why so? Just as there are a variety of foodstuffs that benefit the brain, there are some that have the potential to harm it and most of them—particularly the toxic insults from metals, pesticides, and other chemicals—accumulate over time in small increments that ultimately cause trouble. Just as research has shown that building the most robust brain possible in the early years correlates with a fitter, more active, healthier brain in later years, so does the relative absence of toxic load. The freer your brain tissue remains of the buildup of damaging toxins throughout life, the better the outlook for your brain as it ages. And that means avoiding or at least reducing exposure to some substances. Let's take a look at what you can do.

TRANS-FATS

Avoid trans-fats, which are found mainly in partially hydrogenated vegetable oils, margarine products, and vegetable shortening and are used extensively in food processing.

Trans-fats are a techno-product of food manufacturing, created in the factory laboratory by altering the chemical structure of the polyunsaturated fats found naturally in small amounts in corn, soybeans, and vegetables to make them behave more like saturated fats in baking and food processing. The altered structural properties of trans-fats prevent them from going rancid or spoiling the way natural polyunsaturates would. This feature prolongs their shelf life, whether in a bottle or as a component of prepackaged convenience foods. They pose a brain (and general health) hazard chiefly because they become woven into cell membranes, causing an increase in stiffness that prevents the membrane from functioning properly. They are especially bad news for an organ, such as the brain, that is mostly made of fat. Products containing trans-fats also have an adverse effect on blood lipids; they lower HDL cholesterol and raise low-density lipoproteins, the bad cholesterol.

It's tough to avoid them entirely, because they're so prevalent in today's food supply; however, you can (and should) reduce your intake by cooking with and eating fresh whole foods whenever possible and limiting your intake of prepackaged convenience foods in which trans-fats abound. In addition, avoid consuming margarine; vegetable shortening; and partially hydrogenated corn, vegetable, soybean, safflower, sunflower, and cottonseed oils—whether they come in bottles, tubs, or junk food (check the labels!).

CONCENTRATED SWEETS

Avoid the regular use of concentrated sweets. Large quantities of sugar, corn syrup, and high-fructose corn syrup offer nothing to the brain in the way of nutrition and actively destabilize blood sugar regulation, adding strain to the system and predisposing to memory decline. That is not to say you should vow never to eat another gooey dessert or drink a soda for the rest of your life, which although it would be beneficial to health would prove a tough vow to keep. Rather you should be aware of the high cost of concentrated sweets to your brain. Use sweets in moderation as occasional treats, not in lieu of real food or as daily fare.

FLAVOR ENHANCERS AND ARTIFICIAL SWEETENERS

Avoid monosodium glutamate (MSG), the flavor enhancer used in many processed foods and often in Chinese restaurants, and foods that contain it. Research has indicated it acts as an excitotoxin that causes damage by "exciting" brain cells to death.

Aspartame is a non-nutritive sweetener. Although it appears fairly safe, there are reports of headache, migraine aura, dizziness, confusion, and possibly depressive symptoms related to its use. One double-blind study in childhood epilepsy patients documented a statistically significant increase in seizure duration/frequency. Well-documented instances of thrombocytopenia (low platelet counts) and Sjogren's syndrome related to aspartame consumption appear in the medical literature. For these reasons, I would recommend avoiding its use.

Sucralose, marketed under the brand name Splenda, is a recent arrival to the marketplace. I feel this is also fairly safe although I have heard anecdotal evidence from people who attribute headaches and stomach distress to sucralose consumption. Studies and experience with long-term use are not yet available so even if you appear to tolerate it well, I would still recommend caution.

PESTICIDES, HORMONES, AND ANTIBIOTICS

Avoid consuming brain toxic chemicals. Again, because the brain is mostly made of fat and because many chemicals are soluble in fat, the brain is especially vulnerable to toxins such as heavy metals, pesticides, herbicides, and hormones present in foods. To reduce your exposure, try the following suggestions.

Buy organic produce when possible. Doing so will sharply reduce your exposure to toxic residues from pesticides and herbicides that remain with the food, even after you wash it with soap and water. Some crops tend to be more heavily sprayed than others. For pesticide-heavy foods, it probably makes good brain sense to spend the extra dollars from your food budget to go organic, even if you can't always buy everything organic from your local farmers' market or grocer (see Box 4.1).

Buy organic dairy products. If cows graze on pastures sprayed with pes-

---

BOX 4.1. **Produce with the Most Pesticide Residues***

Apples	Nectarines	Sweet bell peppers
Celery	Peaches	Peaches
Cherries	Spinach	Pears
Grapes (imported)	Strawberries	Potatoes
Lettuce		

*Data from Environmental Working Group "Shopper's Guide to Pesticides in Produce," available at www.foodnews.org (accessed March 2007).

ticides and herbicides or if they are treated with bovine growth hormone, antibiotics, or other chemicals, those substances can appear in the milk. Pesticides, herbicides, hormones, and antibiotics concentrate in the fat of animals, including milk fat. (Nursing mothers should also remember that the same phenomenon occurs in human breast milk.) The alternative, of course, is to drink only fat-free dairy; however, if you love the richness of butter and cream, spend a bit of your food budget on organic dairy products.

Buy organic, natural, or pastured beef, pork, lamb, and poultry for the same reason as organic dairy—the toxins, if present, will concentrate in the fat of the animals. And in this case, there is no fat-free alternative; even boneless, skinless chicken breast contains some fat. The most toxin-free meat comes from animals not given hormones, antibiotics, and growth factors and not fed pesticide-tainted corn or feed. Again, it's a good place to spend food budget dollars if you can.

The Brain-Friendly Plate: Menu Plans

So what does a brain-friendly diet entail? Let's take a look at 1 week of menus from the Brain Trust Program. Remember that what you're aiming to do is incorporate brain-friendly foods into your diet, not restrict your diet to only these foods. Your basic goal in feeding your brain right is to enjoy a varied diet that relies mainly on real food.

These meal plans should give you a good start for planning your own brain-friendly meals. Be inventive, be creative, and try to eat a wide selection of fresh whole foods, including those listed here, every day. You'll soon be on your way to building (or rebuilding) an optimally functioning, healthy brain!

DAY 1

Breakfast

Omelet (1–2 whole eggs plus 1–2 egg whites with butter-sautéed spinach and garlic)

2–3 slices crisp bacon (or turkey bacon)

$1/2$ cup fresh (or frozen) mixed berries

Coffee (decaf or regular) or tea (green, black, herbal)

Lunch

Open-faced tuna and cheese melt (1 slice multigrain bread, homemade tuna salad, and 1 slice Swiss or Cheddar cheese; toast under the broiler)

Garden salad (spinach and lettuces, chopped tomato, carrot, and cucumber with olive oil vinaigrette and a sprinkling of toasted sesame seeds)

1 medium orange

Coffee or tea (green, black, or herbal), as desired

Snack Option

1–2 ounces raw or roasted pumpkin seeds

Dinner

5 ounces broiled salmon (top with butter, lemon, garlic, and dill)

$2/3$ cup broccoli (sauté in sesame oil with garlic, salt, pepper, and sesame seeds)

$1/2$ cup roasted beets (top with a drizzle of pumpkin oil, salt, and pepper)

$1/2$ cup fresh (or frozen) blueberries (top with a dollop of whipping cream)

1 glass light-bodied red wine, if desired

Coffee (decaf or regular) or tea (green, black, herbal)

DAY 2

Breakfast

²/₃ cup plain yogurt (top with fresh or frozen mixed berries and walnuts or pecans; stir in 1–2 scoops of strawberry or vanilla whey protein powder, if desired)

Coffee (decaf or regular) or tea (green, black, herbal)

Lunch

2 stuffed avocado halves (stuff with homemade shrimp salad; serve on a bed of spinach; top with olive oil vinaigrette)

String cheese

3 sesame rice crackers with butter

Coffee (decaf or regular) or tea (green, black, herbal)

Snack Option

8–10 red grapes and 3–6 cheese cubes

Dinner

1 broiled or grilled lamb chop (brush with butter mixed with chopped fresh rosemary, thyme, garlic, and mint)

²/₃ cup roasted red and yellow peppers (drizzle with pumpkin oil or olive oil)

²/₃ cup spinach (sauté in olive oil and garlic; top with a sprinkle of sesame seeds)

1 glass full-bodied red wine, if desired

Coffee (decaf or regular) or tea (green, black, herbal)

DAY 3

Breakfast

2–3 scrambled eggs (with lox, cream cheese, and capers)

Half an everything (multiseed topped) bagel with butter

$1/2$ cup fresh (or frozen) strawberries

Coffee (decaf or regular) or tea (green, black, herbal)

Lunch

Chef's salad (dark greens and lettuces with diced carrot, tomato, cucumber, sliced mushrooms, diced turkey and/or ham, and sliced hard-boiled egg; sprinkle with sunflower seeds and shredded cheese and top with olive oil vinaigrette)

3 Blue Diamond Nut Thin crackers with butter

Coffee (decaf or regular) or tea (green, black, herbal)

Snack Option

6–8 Blue Diamond Nut Thin crackers with almond or peanut butter

Dinner

6 ounces beef kebabs (beef cubes with yellow bell pepper chunks, quartered onions, cherry tomatoes, and zucchini chunks)

$1/2$ cup wild rice pilaf (wild rice mixed with minced garlic and onion sautéed in olive oil; top with slivered almonds and chopped fresh parsley)

Arugula and spinach salad (with sliced tomatoes and pumpkin seed oil vinaigrette)

1 glass of full-bodied red wine, if desired

$1/2$ cup fresh (or frozen) mixed berries (top with a dollop of whipping cream)

Coffee (decaf or regular) or tea (green, black, herbal)

DAY 4

Breakfast

1 cup steel-cut oatmeal (top with fresh berries, chopped walnuts, butter, and a drizzle of honey or 1 packet stevia, if preferred)

2–3 slices crisp bacon (or turkey bacon)

Coffee (decaf or regular) or tea (green, black, herbal)

Lunch

Salmon salad wrap (⅔ cup cooked or canned salmon, diced celery, pickle, mayo, and mustard; place on a lettuce-lined, whole-wheat tortilla; top with a flourish of broccoli sprouts)

Sliced fresh tomato (top with a splash of vinegar and drizzle of olive oil)

1 whole peach

Coffee (decaf or regular) or tea (green, black, herbal)

Snack Option

1–2 ounces trail mix (equal parts pumpkin seeds, almonds, sunflower seeds, cashews, and dried cranberries)

Dinner

6 ounces roast pork tenderloin or chops (brush with olive oil and sprinkle with garlic, sage, rosemary, salt, and pepper)

¾ cup roasted butternut squash (dress with a drizzle of melted butter and sprinkle with cinnamon, nutmeg, salt, and pepper)

½ cup steamed whole green beans (top with a drizzle of pumpkin seed oil, salt, pepper, and garlic powder)

1 glass light-bodied red wine, if desired

Several sliced red plums (sauté in butter, drizzle with honey, sprinkle with toasted coconut and pine nuts)

Coffee (decaf or regular) or tea (green, black, herbal)

DAY 5

Breakfast

1 poached egg (serve atop nests of sautéed fresh spinach and Canadian bacon slices)

1 slice multigrain toast with butter

$1/2$ cup fresh (or frozen) blueberries

Coffee (decaf or regular) or tea (green, black, herbal)

Lunch

Grilled chicken lettuce wraps (4 ounces grilled chicken with diced tomato, cucumber, avocado, and shredded carrots; top with buttermilk ranch dressing; wrap, burrito style, in large crunchy lettuce leaves)

6–8 Blue Diamond Nut Thin crackers with butter

1 red plum

Coffee (decaf or regular) or tea (green, black, herbal)

Snack Option

8–10 black or red grapes and 1–2 ounces string cheese

Dinner

Broiled/grilled lamb burger patties (6 ounces ground lamb with finely diced onion, chopped fresh parsley and mint, salt, and pepper)

$1/2$ cup jazzed-up couscous (seasoned cooked couscous with pine nuts, sautéed onion and garlic, and fresh chopped parsley and mint)

Salad (greens, diced fresh tomatoes, and cucumbers; dress with yogurt dressing—plain yogurt, splash of vinegar, salt, pepper, dash of ground coriander, garlic powder, and finely chopped mint)

1 glass full-bodied red wine, if desired

Coffee (decaf or regular) or tea (green, black, herbal)

DAY 6

Breakfast

Banana-berry smoothie (1 cup each water, plain yogurt, and frozen mixed berries; half a banana, and 1–2 scoops of strawberry protein powder, if desired)

Lunch

Egg salad sandwich (1 chopped hard-boiled egg, dill pickle, black olive, mayo, and mustard; serve with fresh spinach leaves on multigrain bread or whole-wheat tortilla)

$^2/_3$ cup Greek salad (chopped tomatoes, cucumbers, feta, and olives; sprinkle with olive oil, vinegar, salt, and pepper)

$^1/_2$ cup black or red grapes

Coffee (decaf or regular) or tea (green, black, herbal)

Snack Option

4 slices of dry salami, 2 slices of Cheddar cheese, and dill pickle spears

Dinner

6 ounces pan-seared or grilled tuna steak (marinate in olive oil; soy sauce; pepper; and minced fresh ginger, garlic, rosemary, thyme, and parsley)

1 cup mixed vegetables (sauté zucchini, carrot, yellow squash, and eggplant chunks and garlic in olive oil; season with salt and pepper)

$^1/_2$ cup nutty wild rice (wild rice with sliced almonds, chopped pecans, and sautéed onion; top with chopped fresh cilantro, if desired)

1 glass light-bodied red wine, if desired

Coffee (decaf or regular) or tea (green, black, herbal)

DAY 7

Breakfast

3 ounces ham and 1 ounce cheese omelet (top with salsa and slices of avocado)

1 slice multigrain toast with butter

$1/2$ cup blackberries

Coffee (decaf or regular) or tea (green, black, herbal)

Lunch

Chicken salad wrap ($1/2$ cup diced cooked chicken, red grape halves, diced celery, sliced almonds, mayo, salt, pepper, and chopped fresh parsley; wrap in a lettuce-lined, whole-wheat tortilla)

1 fresh red or purple plum

Coffee (decaf or regular) or tea (green, black, herbal)

Sanck Option

$1/2$ apple and 1 hard-boiled egg

Dinner

6 ounces shrimp or chicken curry (sauté meat in sesame oil with garlic, onion, and red curry paste; add frozen green peas, coconut milk, salt, and pepper)

Baked banana (drizzle with butter, cinnamon, and nutmeg)

2 Grilled red plum halves (brush with olive oil; grill briefly over high heat; drizzle with balsamic vinegar)

1 glass light- to medium-bodied red wine, if desired

Coffee (decaf or regular) or tea (green, black, herbal)

5

Supplemental Nutrition for the Brain: What (and What Not) to Take

If you ate a perfect diet, would you need to take supplemental nutrients to ensure you'd have a healthy, quickly responsive brain and an excellent memory? Possibly not, at least in theory. But odds are that, if you're like most Americans, you don't eat a perfect diet. Few of us eat a diet so rich and varied that, absent supplementing a bit of this or that, we lack for nothing, that our brains have all and more of any nutrient we might need to perform optimally. Even fewer of us eat a diet so pure that it's devoid of any trace of chemical preservative, growth factor, antibiotic, pesticide, toxin, hormone, or molecule of trans-fat, which over time, might do us—and our brains—harm.

Through a lifetime of less than perfect nutrition and exposure to toxic insults, large and small, a brain accumulates a portfolio of dings and dents that cause it to deteriorate; like a priceless antique car, the older a brain gets, the more effort and upkeep it requires to keep it looking sharp and running smoothly. This process of deterioration—medically termed *neurodegenera-tion*—leads ultimately to the weakening of contact points through which brain and nerve cells communicate with one another to store memories, to learn, to transmit thoughts, and to translate thoughts into actions.

With enough accumulated damage, the cells will decay and die. Granted, it doesn't happen overnight. The process starts slowly, almost imperceptibly, like the melting of an ice cube, but it speeds up as time passes and the number of dings mounts up. If we don't intervene by providing good nutrition, including supplemental nutrients, symptoms will eventually appear. Wherever you fall on the spectrum of brain health, I recommend supplementing with at least a few brain-critical nutrients. Research shows that it's never too late to start or, for that matter, never too early either.

I designed this supplement regimen for optimal brain health to work in concert with a brain healthy diet of wholesome foods, not as a substitute for it. I strongly recommend taking certain supplemental nutrients as a means of achieving your brain's peak performance and ensuring its nutritional safety, but I encourage you to think of these supplements as being like seat belts. Just as wearing a seat belt can improve your odds of surviving a collision but won't keep you from having one if you drive recklessly, the best and most effective nutritional supplements in the world can't make up for eating a poor-quality diet, smoking, drinking to excess, being a couch potato, or engaging in high-risk-of-head-injury behaviors.

I recommend that everyone following the Brain Trust Program take certain nutritional supplements to enhance their basic healthy diet. Here's what, how much, and why.

Functional Fats: Marine Lipids and Krill Oil

As you learned in Chapter 4, the brain relies heavily on the delicate essential fats that make up so much of its structure and are critical for brain cell function. An ideal human diet would contain a nearly equal balance of polyunsaturated fats of the omega-6 and omega-3 types. Unfortunately, the modern diet is so weighted toward the omega-6 fatty acids—because of our heavy reliance on vegetable oils (such as corn, safflower, and cottonseed oil)—that what should be a 1:1 or at most a 2:1 ratio of omega-6 to omega-3 fatty acids has tilted to a 20:1 or even 30:1 ratio. This sharply skewed imbalance favors inflammation and robs the brain of the types of fats it needs to function well, those being primarily eicosapentanoic acid (EPA) and docosahexanoic acid (DHA).

EPA and DHA are essential for the building of the brain and brain extensions, such as the eyes (particularly the retina, the seeing structure at the back of the eye that contains the rich collection of nerve endings that connect directly to the brain), in the developing child, both in the womb and in early life, making them critical nutrients for the pregnant or nursing mother. But all of us, from before our birth and throughout our lives, require these fats for the ongoing repair and maintenance of brain and sensory organs, especially the eyes. It's an added benefit that the omega-3 fatty acids also help lower triglyceride levels and reduce inflammation, issues that take on special importance as we age.

Although you can certainly eat more cold-water fish to tip the balance back toward an omega ratio more favorable for the brain, that avenue carries with it a slightly increased toxic burden from the bad stuff that can also be stored in the fat of the fish alongside the omega-3s. Because of the potential for environmental contamination, fish oil is one, and perhaps the best, example of why taking a supplement may be a safer and better alternative than getting the nutrient solely from food. Nowhere is this advice truer than for the developing brain of a child who is nursing or still in the womb; the brains of fetuses, infants, and young children are exquisitely sensitive to mercury and other heavy-metal toxins. Consequently, I especially recommend that pregnant women and nursing mothers limit their intake of fish and instead use a quality fish oil preparation as their primary source of added DHA and EPA.

Reputable manufacturers of pure fish oil preparations use a method called molecular distillation to remove heavy metals such as mercury as well as pesticides, polychlorinated biphenyls (PCBs), dioxins, furans, and other assorted pollutants that find their way into the fat stores of fish. Some manufacturers even bypass the fish entirely and have developed techniques to harvest their omega-3 fatty acids directly from algae farmed in a controlled environment, which eliminates the possibility of toxic contaminants in the first place.

When you purchase a fish oil product, you should be certain that the manufacturer states that the product is free of toxic compounds (look for wording such as "molecularly distilled") and that it is tested for purity and for the presence of rancid (oxidized) fats, preferably by an independent third party.

Recommended dosage: 1–2 grams per day

Recommended form: Molecularly distilled EPA/DHA omega-3 mixture

KRILL OIL

You might rather choose to take krill oil instead of standard fish oil, and here's why. As a general rule of thumb, small fish get eaten by bigger fish who get eaten by bigger fish still, meaning that, usually, the bigger the fish, the higher it is on the food chain and the greater the opportunity for all the toxins and metals from the fish it's eaten to be concentrated in its fat. One large exception is some species of whales, which, despite their enormous size, feast mainly on krill.

Krill, tiny shrimp-like creatures, inhabit the lowest rung of the food ladder, dining mainly on plankton, which are the actual omega-3 factories. As a result, krill enjoy a low risk of being contaminated by the mercury or other toxins present in their larger fishy cousins. In addition, they are a renewable resource; krill represent the largest biomass in the ocean, and there is no risk of endangerment from over harvesting. Their oil, in my opinion, is the best source of essential brain fats available. Not only does krill oil provide substantial amounts of EPA and DHA but it also contains a rich supply of another group of critical fatty substances necessary for brain and nerve cell membranes to function properly: the phospholipids, which play important roles in signal transmission, in energy generation, and in the construction of the insulation coating myelin (which helps speed conduction along the brain's communication pathways). The omega-3 fatty acids in krill oil are bound to these phospholipids. This unique relationship greatly facilitates the passage of the fatty acid molecules through your intestinal wall making them much more bioavailable (easily incorporated by the body). The predominant phospholipid in krill oil is phosphatidylcholine, making it a rich source of choline, which many studies have demonstrated as being important in brain development, learning, and memory. It is also the precursor for the vital memory neurotransmitter acetylcholine.

Krill oil also naturally contains high concentrations of a number of healthy antioxidant compounds that not only protect the krill oil but also protect your brain when you consume it. These include vitamin A, vitamin E, astaxanthin, and canthaxanthin. Astaxanthin forms a special linkage with EPA and DHA, thus making it more readily available to the body than other antioxidants on the market. For this reason, while consumption of fish oil breaks down and therefore decreases your body's antioxidant concentrations, krill oil actually increases levels of antioxidants in the body.

One last bit of advice: Don't store your krill oil in the refrigerator; which will make the gel caps weep and stick together. Just keep them in a cool, dry, dark place.

Recommended dosage: 2–4 capsules per day

Recommended form: Antarctic pure Neptuno Krill Oil

The B Vitamin Group

The B vitamins—thiamin (B_1), riboflavin (B_2), niacin (B_3), pyridoxine (B_6), cobalamin (B_{12}), folic acid, pantothenic acid, biotin, and choline—make up a family of nutrients that plays fundamental roles in the functioning of the nervous system. Although these vitamins have important functions throughout the body, such as reducing homocysteine and decreasing the risk for heart disease and stroke, their critical nervous system and brain-related tasks range from driving energy-generating pathways to balancing hormone levels to helping manufacture neurotransmitters (chemical-signaling messengers) such as acetylcholine.

Vitamin B_{12} and folate are necessary for the formation of myelin. Deficiency of these two players in the adult can result in severe weakness, loss of mental function, and depression of mind and motion and—if left uncorrected—can lead to memory loss and even frank dementia. Deficiency that occurs in a developing fetus can result in birth defects such as spina bifida, a failure of the spinal canal to close properly during its development that often results in pronounced weakness or actual paralysis of the legs. For this reason alone, it is absolutely mandatory that pregnant women must be sure to get plenty of B vitamins, particularly folate (also called folic acid) each day throughout pregnancy.

Unfortunately, the typical American diet doesn't always provide adequate amounts of these vital nutrients, which, since they are water soluble and therefore not stored, must be present in the diet every day. Moreover, the very people who would be most at risk for decline in mental function and memory loss—the elderly and those with chronic illnesses—are the groups most likely to eat a diet deficient in B vitamins, both because this group generally eats fewer calories from a more restricted range of foods and because they may have trouble absorbing the nutrients from what they do eat. For these groups especially, but for anyone concerned about preserving, restoring, or improving brain function and memory, I recommend supplementation with a B vitamin complex containing the whole family.

Recommended dosage: thiamin 20 milligrams, riboflavin 20 milligrams, niacin 20 milligrams, pantothenic acid 20 milligrams, biotin 300 micrograms, pyridoxine (B_6) 20 milligrams, cobalamin (B_{12}) 100 micrograms, folic acid 800 micrograms, and choline 20 milligrams

Recommended form: Use the niacinamide or nicotinamide form of the B vitamin niacin if possible; these forms cross into the brain four times better than any other form

Magnesium

The unsung hero of the nutrient world is, without a doubt, magnesium. Although a critical cofactor required for more than 300 different chemical reactions in the body, this essential element often gets thought of as little more than the poor relation of the darling of the media, calcium. Because magnesium isn't plentiful in many foods (dark green leafy vegetables and nuts, excepted), it has no strong lobby to ask us regularly, "Got magnesium?" And yet, the biochemical relationship between magnesium and its glory-hogging cousin is at the very crux of preserving memory and brain health.

As you have learned in detail in Chapter 2, a tightly orchestrated flow of calcium into the nerve cells must occur in just the right amount and at just the correct moment for a brain or nerve signal (which could involve a thought, a memory, or an action) to fire. No calcium entry, no firing. The paradox, however, is that the very same calcium molecule, so critical for the brain cell to work, carries with it a deadly potential. The brain or nerve cell opens the door (or calcium channel as it's called) to hustle the calcium in and then shoves it back out the door when it's done its work. If calcium builds up inside the brain cell, it will overstimulate it and may ultimately destroy it.

Pharmaceutical giants have spent many millions (perhaps even billions) of dollars developing drugs that slow down the entry of calcium into cells without blocking the flow entirely, which would obviously result in no firing at all and be counterproductive. The results of this quest by the drug makers has been the development of the calcium channel blocker class of drugs for blood pressure in the cardiovascular arena and drugs such as memantine (Namenda) in the area of memory as treatments for those people suffering with Alzheimer's disease. Memantine is a weak calcium channel blocker that, while pretty safe, still has an extensive profile of side effects and adverse reactions listed in its bio.

What does all this have to do with magnesium? Magnesium is nature's own weak calcium channel blocker, able to put the brakes on excessive flow of calcium ions into the brain or nerve cells, but without the potential for side effects and at substantially less cost. Science bears its efficacy out; research has demonstrated that magnesium supplementation improved memory and other troublesome symptoms in patients with dementia. The results aren't really so surprising, because magnesium exerts its effect on the calcium channel in much the same way that memantine does, but with an added bonus: magnesium not only slows down the degree of brain/nerve cell excitement by calcium flow but also acts to increase the forces within the cell that offset excitement, leading to a better balance between these opposing forces. This inhibition of excitement may in part account for its ability to relax tight muscles and facilitate restful sleep. It's also what makes it an ideal nutrient to protect the delicate nerve endings in the ears involved with both the sense of hearing and of balance. Supplemental magnesium acts to protect against noise-induced hearing loss from the inside like protective gear helps externally—a connection that should prove of great benefit to today's generation of iPod-toting teens.

Magnesium causes very few of what you could call side effects. However, some forms of it aren't well absorbed and can lead to diarrhea by promoting increased water content in the bowels and softer stools. Because of this action in the body, Milk of Magnesia is a well-known over-the-counter remedy for constipation. For those troubled by constipation, this side effect can actually be a major benefit. People not so afflicted, however, can avoid diarrhea by selecting a chelated form of magnesium instead of a less well absorbed form such as magnesium oxide, and then working up to a level of tolerance slowly.

Recommended dosage: 600 milligrams (elemental magnesium) taken alone, if possible, at bedtime; if necessary work up to this dosage (begin with 200 milligrams for a few weeks, advance to 400 milligrams, and then to 600 milligrams as intestinal tolerance permits)

Recommended form: magnesium chelate (magnesium malate or complexed as magnesium taurinate)

Taurine

Taurine is a naturally occurring sulfur-containing amino acid that plays key roles in the development and well-being of brain and nerve cells. First isolated from the bile of oxen (hence the name, derived from Taurus, the bull) and found in meat and other animal proteins, taurine is classified as a conditionally essential amino acid (related to the amount of meat that is consumed) for humans who eat meat, fish, poultry, and eggs. Vegans, who choose not to eat any animal protein, need to consider taurine as a fully essential amino acid because it occurs only in trace amounts in plant foods. This means taurine must be added to the diet, usually in supplement form, because humans don't make taurine as well as most other mammals. Cats don't make taurine at all. Without taurine in their diet, cats will suffer degeneration of the retinal tissues in the back of the eye and become blind.

Unlike other amino acids, taurine is never incorporated into large body proteins, such as those that make up muscle, but instead occurs free in the bloodstream and tissues, including the brain. In the brain, its primary action is to exert a relaxing effect that offers a counterbalance to overexcitement brought on by too much calcium. Taurine steps in when an excess of calcium flows into the brain cell or when exposure to excitotoxic compounds, such as monosodium glutamate (MSG), leads to calcium overload. A sudden rise in calcium within the cell spurs a release of taurine, which acts like a fire extinguisher to quiet the riot and protect the cell from damage. Taurine and magnesium work as a team to balance overstimulation of nerve cells.

Research has shown that taurine levels are low in people with Alzheimer's disease and in those with diabetes; in the first case, possibly contributing to memory decline and, in the second, contributing to stroke risk by making the blood platelets stickier and the blood more likely to clot. Supplementation appears to raise the level of free taurine in the blood and in the fluid that surrounds the brain, which research has shown, at least in the case of the platelets, is able to reverse the defect and render them less sticky. Less sticky platelets means less likelihood of a blood clot and also means lower risk for stroke, which, of course, is a good thing for preserving your brain. In the case of memory, research in animals indicates that adding taurine to the diet increases brain levels of acetylcholine (ACH), the most critical neurotransmitter involved in memory. As ACH levels fall, memory fails. Making more ACH available to the brain's communication network improves memory, and intriguing research suggests that taurine may help do just that.

Recommended dosage: 1 gram each morning and 1 gram each evening

Recommended form: taurine as the free amino acid

Acetyl L-Carnitine

Carnitine is an amino acid found in high amounts in meat; it takes its name from the same root word (*carne*, "flesh") as *carnivorous*, meaning "meat eating." Plain carnitine acts chiefly in the body in the energy-production department, oiling the wheels of the shuttle mechanism that ferries fats into the mitochondria (the powerhouse furnaces within each cell of the body), where they are burned for energy.

Acetyl L-carnitine (ALC), is a variation of plain carnitine with a chemical attachment (the acetyl group) that makes it particularly useful to the brain and nervous system and for that matter for the heart as well, proving once again that what's good for the heart is good for the brain. Just as it does throughout the body, the carnitine part of ALC serves to drive fat molecules efficiently into the energy furnaces to boost energy production. The acetyl part then becomes available to promote the manufacturing of that all-important memory messenger, *acetyl*choline, which, as you've learned, is needed for both the storage of new memories and the retrieval of older ones.

Intriguing research in rats and people suggests that as the levels of ACH begin to decline with age (or disease) and as memory begins to falter, supplementation of the diet with ALC may boost ACH levels and improve short-term and long-term memory, increase attention span and focus, and improve hand–eye coordination and reaction speed. Other studies suggest that ALC improves verbal fluency and spatial memory. And the benefits aren't limited to just the older population. In one study involving women aged 22 to 27, supplemental ALC for a 30-day period caused large increases in speed of learning, speed of reaction, and reduction of errors on complex visual tests.

But beyond its roles in energy provisioning and memory boosting, ALC also offers protective benefits to the brain cells. It works to keep a lid on free-radical production, which protects the delicate fats in the brain from being damaged by oxygen and, in a word, going rancid. ALC also appears to retard the age-related drop in nerve growth factors, such as brain-derived neurotrophic factor (BDNF), which helps rebuild new brain and nerve tissues. In addition, in structures that deteriorate over time, such as the myelin sheath,

ALC appears to slow and perhaps even reverse the degenerative process—at least in mice.

Several controlled human studies, primarily in patients with age-related memory decline, Alzheimer's disease, and Parkinson's disease, have been completed, and others are under way to assess the value of this simple amino acid variant as a serious treatment option in these diseases. So far, ALC appears to be one of the few substances that can slow down the progression of Alzheimer's disease. I strongly recommend that anyone concerned about preserving or improving mental function take ALC.

Recommended dosage: 100–500 milligrams (1,500–2,000 milligrams have been used experimentally in Alzheimer's and Parkinson's disease trials without serious side effects)

Recommended form: as pure acetyl L-carnitine

α-Lipoic Acid

Everybody's heard that antioxidants are important for health; they fight free-radicals, help keep the skin younger, protect our eyes from the damaging rays of the sun, and may even prevent some types of cancer. Ask 20 people on a busy city street anywhere in America what the most important antioxidant for good health might be and you're sure to get a variety of answers: β-carotene, vitamin C, and vitamin E; maybe a few will offer coenzyme Q10 (CoQ_{10}). But virtually nobody would come up with α-lipoic acid. And yet, in the supplemental nutrient world, there is quite possibly no more versatile or important antioxidant, chiefly because, in a manner of speaking, it gets along with everybody.

For antioxidants to do their work—neutralizing the harmful effects of free-radicals, for instance—they must take the fight to the neighborhood where the free-radicals breed and thrive. For the most part, this means in and around the energy-generating powerhouses, or mitochondria. Sounds simple enough, but it's not, because some antioxidants can't get there. Many (such as vitamin C and β-carotene) can dissolve in water but are repelled by oil and fat. Others (such as CoQ_{10}) can dissolve in oil and fat but not in water. α-lipoic acid—or thioctic acid, as it's sometimes called—dissolves readily in either, an attribute that gives it a major advantage over its antioxidant kin in getting to where the free-radicals live. Here's why.

The outside surface of every cell (or for that matter every mitochondrion or other intracellular compartment) in the body is a membrane or shell that allows the cell to carefully control what comes in and what stays out. It is a fatty shell that encloses the watery interior of the cell. Because oil and water don't mix, it is difficult for fat-soluble antioxidants to move around in the watery portion and for water-soluble antioxidants to get through the fatty cell membrane. Being a switch hitter in the game of solubility, α-lipoic acid can easily navigate through both the fatty outer layer and the watery inner portion of the cell. It can even take its free-radical-quenching power straight through to the mitochondria themselves, where most of the free-radicals arise.

Although α-lipoic acid is naturally manufactured in small amounts in the body, its production declines as we age, an unfortunate circumstance, indeed, because we need it all the more as we get older. The need becomes even greater for those of us who suffer with insulin resistance or diabetes, since research indicates that α-lipoic acid helps control blood sugar and may thus help prevent some of the complications of that disease on the brain and elsewhere. Emerging research suggests that α-lipoic acid may even help *delay* the onset of diabetes in the first place, which, as you've already learned is important to brain health.

A chief cause of diabetic complications comes from a simple chemical reaction that occurs when sugar in the blood, brain, or other tissues irreversibly attaches to and permanently alters proteins in the body. The process, called *glycation*, results in visible or obvious damage throughout the body; everything from age spots on the skin to cataracts in the eyes. Less obvious damage occurs, particularly in people with diabetes, to nerves throughout the body, causing numbness, weakness, and pain, a condition called *peripheral neuropathy*. Physicians in Europe regularly use hefty doses (300 to 600 milligrams per day) of α-lipoic acid to treat patients suffering from this disorder, and patients often see improvement in their symptoms in as little as 3 weeks. Some research scientists have even documented nerve regeneration in patients with diabetes who were treated with high-dose α-lipoic acid therapy.

Supplementation with α-lipoic acid in this dosing range should be done only under the guidance of a health-care practitioner because it may, albeit rarely, produce low blood sugar.

The benefits of α-lipoic acid for nerve tissues don't end there; at the other end of peripheral nerves lies the brain. Because α-lipoic acid can easily cross the blood–brain barrier, a semipermeable protective membrane surrounding the brain, it can gain entry into the brain cells, where it also serves to protect their delicate fats from oxidizing and becoming rancid. One recent study, done in mice, bears this out. Researchers supplemented aging mice with α-lipoic acid and discovered that it enhanced their spatial memory (demonstrated by how well they can remember how to run through a maze). Some of the mice performed the task as well as mice half their age. The scientists speculate that boosting the antioxidant effect in the brain tissue of the mice with α-lipoic acid protected the animals' brain cells and better preserved the cell-to-cell connection networks, thus enhancing memory. We're not mice, of course, but the result is spawning promising human trials that may soon help explain why α-lipoic acid seems to be so good for the human brain.

Unfortunately, we can't simply rely on food intake to provide us with a sufficient amount of this nutritious compound, since there are few good food sources of it. It is amazing that when it was first discovered, in 1937, researchers needed 10 tons of beef liver to extract just 30 milligrams of the stuff. Although one of the richest food sources is spinach, we would have to eat about 7 pounds of spinach to get just 1 milligram of α-lipoic acid. Here, more than with any other brain critical nutrient, the miracles of modern technology come to the rescue with good supplemental sources.

Recommended dosage: 50–300 milligrams daily

Recommended form: any reputable brand

Coenzyme Q10

Coenzyme Q10 is a fat- or oil-soluble antioxidant found in the cellular membranes and within the interior of every one of the trillions of cells in the body, hence its other name, *ubiquinone*, derived from the same Latin root as is the word *ubiquitous*, meaning "everywhere." Its highest concentrations, however, occur in the mitochondria found in the most metabolically active tissues, such as the brain, heart, kidneys, and liver, where it serves both as a powerful defender against oxidation and free-radicals and as a key player in energy production.

CoQ_{10} has long been the subject of study as a potential treatment for such degenerative disorders of the brain and nerves as Alzheimer's disease, Parkinson's disease, and amyotrophic lateral sclerosis (ALS), or Lou Gehrig's disease. Laboratory research has shown that when investigators supplemented the diets of mice with CoQ_{10} before giving them a substance toxic to their mitochondria, the mice suffered less nerve and brain damage. In other words, the CoQ_{10} seemed to offer significant protection from a severe toxic insult.

Although we can get some CoQ_{10} from foods such as salmon, liver, and other organ meats, it's almost impossible to get enough from diet alone. The body does make CoQ_{10}, in fact using the same key enzyme in the cholesterol production pathway that the statin drugs inhibit. However, as with so many other substances, CoQ_{10} production falls off with age. Therefore, supplementation with this key nutrient is important for anyone who cares about preserving and optimizing brain health. Because the statin drugs block the production of CoQ_{10}, people who take them for cholesterol lowering *must* supplement with CoQ_{10}.

Recommended dosage: 25–100 milligrams per day; 300 milligrams per day for statin users

Recommended form: CoQ_{10} requires oil for absorption into the body, so choose a form encapsulated in an oil base (usually rice bran oil) or one that melts in the mouth on contact with saliva. (if you cannot find a product that meets these criteria, be sure to take your supplement with a meal containing fat or oil)

Vitamin D

Often called the sunshine vitamin because we make it naturally when sunlight acts on cholesterol in our skin, vitamin D could also be called the feel-good vitamin. We now understand that a chemical wizardry occurs when sun meets skin that triggers the brain's production of the feel-good brain chemical serotonin (the same one many prescription antidepressant medications are designed to raise). This effect probably accounts for why getting out in the sunshine makes most of us happier and why sunlight deprivation makes us feel blue.

For some people, the absence of sunlight has a profound effect on mood, causing a condition known as seasonal affective disorder (SAD), in the fall and winter months. Vitamin D may be the link between the sun and the brain that leads to outright depression in this group of people and the winter blahs in the rest of us. Researchers investigated this connection by giving people with SAD 400 or 800 International Units (IU) of vitamin D on each of 5 days in late winter. They discovered it lifted the patients' spirits and made them feel better.

But beyond elevating mood, vitamin D is both a potent antioxidant and an anti-inflammatory agent. In the latter capacity, it protects the brain against the toxic effects of the inflammatory compounds that, sad to say, increase in all of us as we age, but especially so in those with Alzheimer's disease. A rising tide of inflammatory compounds will ultimately disrupt the cell-to-cell communication connections, short-circuit the memory, and, if left unchecked, can even lead to brain cell death. Vitamin D, a fat-soluble vitamin, can readily enter the brain, which you'll recall is made largely of delicate fats. Once there, it can deliver a powerful one-two punch against both inflammation and free-radical oxidation.

Recommended dosage: 400 IU to no more than 2,000 IU per day (note: the body can store vitamin D, making it possible for the vitamin to build up to toxic levels)

Recommended form: vitamin D_3 in oil such as a soft gel

Although it's my firm belief that anyone interested in improving, preserving, or optimizing brain health should supplement daily with at least the minimum amounts suggested for each nutrient discussed to far, there are a few more supplemental nutrients that I'll mention. While the following are not necessary for everyone, they may be important for people specifically concerned about improving memory and focus, whether they're students, harried parents, busy executives, professionals, or older folks.

Huperzine A

Originally a botanical supplement, huperzine is an extract of *Huperzia serrata*, or Chinese club moss, a plant in the fern family reputedly significantly unchanged since prehistoric times. In traditional Chinese medicine, it is called *qian ceng ta* ("thousand-laid pagoda," a term derived from the shape of the plant) or *jin bu huan* ("more valuable than gold"). For centuries, Chinese medical practitioners relied on this plant to treat swelling, fever, and inflammation as well as to enhance memory in the elderly. Although modern clinical trials in China have documented the plant's effectiveness both to combat memory loss with aging and to protect the brain cells against trauma and degeneration, conventional Western medicine has been slow to catch on.

The active ingredient in *jin bu huan*, called huperzine, exists in two forms in the moss: a potent variety denoted as huperzine A and a much weaker one, called huperzine B. Both of these extracts act to prevent the breakdown of the most important brain chemical involved in memory, ACH, in much the same way as do the current prescription medications, such as Aricept, developed to treat Alzheimer's disease. By slowing the breakdown of ACH, huperize allows more ACH to remain available to the communication network in the brain. At the rate that brain cells talk to one another even extending ACH's useful life by a few milliseconds can make a profound difference in memory and focus in young and old alike.

One recent human clinical trial in China found that giving huperzine A to a group of older people suffering from Alzheimer's significantly improved the patients' cognitive (mental) function, mood, behavior, and ability to perform the typical activities of normal daily living. Their caregivers independently confirmed patients who took the supplement made notable improvement in quality of life.

In studies at the other end of the age spectrum, in junior high and middle school students with memory and learning difficulties, huperzine A was again shown in a randomized, double-blind trial to exert a beneficial effect on memory and learning aptitude without noted side effects.

Recent studies have shown that huperzine A also acts as a potent antioxidant and anti-inflammatory agent. In addition, by limiting the flow of calcium ions into brain cells (a topic we explored in Chapter 2), it promotes cell survival and protects against overstimulation and excitotoxicity. In so doing, huperzine A acts in much the same way as Namenda, one of the newest pharmaceutical weapons in the fight to treat Alzheimer's disease, and does so with far less potential for unpleasant or dangerous side effects. It's important to note that because huperzine A slows the breakdown of ACH, people with seizure disorders, heart rhythm disturbances, emphysema, ulcers, or an enlarged prostate should consult with their physicians before taking this supplement.

Dosage recommendation: 75–100 micrograms twice a day for adults; 50 micrograms twice daily for adolescents; only under medical supervision for younger children

Recommended form: Synthetically manufactured supplements are amenable to precise dosing; for Chinese herbal form, the product should be third-party tested to ensure that it contains what it should and is free of heavy-metal contamination

Vinpocetine

I recommend vinpocetine, an extract of the periwinkle plant, *Vinca minor*, especially for the elderly population and those with known atherosclerotic disease (hardening of the arteries) or with other medical conditions known to contribute to artery hardening such as diabetes or insulin resistance syndromes. The process of atherosclerosis can occur throughout the body. Hardening of the arteries in the heart predisposes the patient to heart attack; in the extremities, atherosclerosis can cause muscle cramping and difficulty walking. In the head and neck, the narrowing of arteries by plaque cuts blood flow to a trickle, depriving the brain of sufficient oxygen, glucose, and other nutrients necessary to function properly, so that thinking, reaction speed, and memory decline. Most ominous, hardening of the arteries in the brain also increases the possibility of having a stroke.

Physicians in Europe and Japan have used supplemental vinpocetine for more than 20 years to treat people for conditions caused by inadequate blood flow to the brain. Results from more than 50 clinical studies demonstrate its usefulness in improving blood flow to the brain, promoting better delivery of oxygen and nutrients to the brain, assisting the brain cells in powering themselves more effectively, and even helping prevent the formation of blood clots in tiny arteries.

But the brain benefits of vinpocetine don't stop there. Other healthy attributes, discovered more recently, include a potent antioxidant capability that enhances the power of other antioxidants such as α-lipoic acid; CoQ_{10}; vitamins A, C, and E; and the group of more than 5,000 flavonoid compounds found in fruits, vegetables, and spices. It has also demonstrated an ability to protect brain cells from excessive stimulation, which occurs early on in the cascade of events triggered when blood flow to a section of the brain diminishes markedly.

Although potentially beneficial for all brains, I consider vinpocetine a required nutrient for people with artery narrowing, because I have witnessed remarkable clinical improvement in patients with vascular dementia who have taken the supplement. I would offer one caution, however: Because of its blood thinning action, people who take blood thinners, such as Coumadin, should use vinpocetine only under a doctor's supervision.

Recommended dosage: 5–10 milligrams twice a day

Recommended form: any reputable brand

Because many of us take a daily multivitamin or mineral preparation, we must be careful not to combine nutritional supplements that contain excessive amounts of any of the various components. This frequently requires a carefully orchestrated balancing act to achieve effective amounts of the desired ingredients and not too much of any one of them. If you are taking supplemental nutrients already, especially if they include some of the brain-specific nutrients I have discussed, you must account for what you are currently taking and appropriately adjust dosages to keep everything at the desired amount.

Another approach is to take a brain-specific nutrient product that has been clinically tested and found to be both safe and effective. One possibility is a product I designed and tested called Lucidal (see www.lucidal.com).

In Chapter 7 we investigate some common brain-related disorders, including hot flashes, migraines, and sensory disturbances, and I make specific recommendations for nutrient cocktails, or customized therapies for each condition. Obviously, the amounts of each supplement must be integrated with any products that you will be taking concurrently. This will be explored in more detail in each specific context.

What Not to Take

IRON

Topping the list of what *not* to take is iron. Despite the advertisements by the makers of iron tonic supplements, such as Geritol, that tout their product as a remedy for the fatigue and weakness brought on by iron deficiency, very few people actually need to take supplemental iron. That's not to say that iron isn't important to health, because it absolutely is. Nor do I intend to imply that people with iron deficiency documented by their physicians and by appropriate laboratory tests shouldn't take iron supplements; it's just that most of us don't fall into that category. Men particularly, but also women primarily after menopause, have an abundance of iron stored away. The human body easily absorbs and ferociously hangs on to iron; in fact, once it's inside us, we have no way to get rid of iron, except by blood loss, which is the main way anyone who actually does need iron becomes deficient in it. But why is it a problem?

Iron is a pro-oxidant—that is, a substance that reacts vigorously and easily with oxygen. Consider what happens to an iron hinge or nail left to the mercies of the oxygen in the air. It rusts in short order. Given enough time, even something as huge as the unpainted body of a truck will utterly dissolve into a pile of rust, which is nothing but oxidized iron.

Excess iron is stored throughout the body by a compound doctors call *ferritin*, which can be measured with a simple blood test. Within ferritin packets, iron is relatively harmless; however, stored iron can be set loose into the tissues under certain circumstances (such as a blockage or reduction in blood flow through the arteries.) Once free, iron will react with oxygen in an explosion of oxidation that wreaks havoc wherever it happens, doing to the heart or the brain the same thing it does to the hinge or the truck.

Recommendation: Do not take iron supplements or multivitamin and mineral preparations containing iron *unless* prescribed by your physician to treat documented iron deficiency. If lab tests determine you've stored excess iron, rid yourself of it by controlled bleeding: Give blood at your local blood bank. This may be done once every 56 days.

SUPPLEMENT QUALITY

While this chapter makes it clear that micronutrient supplements are a key part of the Brain Trust Program, my recommendation for taking them comes with a caveat: Beware of cheap sources of nutritional supplements! The quality of a supplement product is only as good as its ingredients and the integrity of its maker. In an industry that is largely unregulated, this point matters. Some manufacturers purchase the cheapest raw ingredients to make their products, particularly for botanical or herbal supplements. China is a common source for these materials. Unfortunately, although they may contain adequate amounts of the active ingredient, many of them also contain unwanted contaminants, such as toxic heavy metals.

A group of investigators in Dallas decided to take a critical look at the reliability of labels on nutritional supplements. They pulled nutritional supplements randomly from the shelves of local Dallas health food stores and evaluated the products to see if they contained what their labels said. The results: A majority of the products didn't contain the active ingredient in the amount listed on the label, some by a little less, some by a lot. And a shocking percentage didn't contain *any measurable amount* of the active ingredient! Lest you think this is something peculiar to Dallas, the products tested were mainly national brands, sold in health food stores all across the country.

Recommendation: Purchase your supplements from a reputable source. Even then, ask if the company submits each of its products to independent third-party testing to ensure purity, quality, and quantity of contents and whether it makes the results of quality assurance testing available. If in doubt, ask to see that documentation.

Now that you're acquainted with what and what not to eat and take, let's turn our attention to what and what not to do as we examine the benefits of appropriate exercise on the brain.

Exercise
for the Brain:
What (and What Not)
to Do

The Greeks knew it nearly 2,500 years ago: *Mens sana in corpore sano,* they told us—"A sound mind in a sound body." They based their understanding of the close connection between mind and body on what they could observe, but modern day science has proven their observations were right on the money. Recent and very exciting scientific research has shown us that those workouts in the gym don't just help you shed unwanted pounds, add pleasing curves in just the right places, and make you feel better but even help you to think better and, more important, help your brain age more gracefully.

Although we're all aware that the lack of physical exercise may raise the risk of developing such disorders as diabetes, heart disease, cancer, and osteoarthritis, we're generally less familiar with a growing body of research evidence that suggests a strong connection between physical activity and preservation of brain function. This includes not only the thinking and reasoning functions but mood as well!

One recent study, for instance, concluded that women who walked more miles per week were more likely to keep their brains sharper as they aged than their sedentary counterparts. Another study followed subjects for 6 years and showed that those people who were the most *physically* fit at the start of the study were the most *mentally* fit 6 years later. Yet another has linked improved levels of focus, attention, and thinking in middle age with level of physical activity at age 36, clearly emphasizing that it's never too early to begin laying the foundation for mental sharpness in later years by becoming physically more fit now.

Modern brain scanning techniques give us a glimpse into the effect of physical training on the brain. Researchers asked a group of older, healthy adults to participate in a 6-month program of aerobic training. Brain scan pictures made after participation in the regimen compared with those made before commencing the training showed an increase in the amount of both gray matter and white matter within the brain. The researchers interpreted these findings as suggesting that the aerobic exercise had not only increased the number of blood vessels supplying oxygen and nutrients throughout the brain and strengthened and beefed up the insulation around the brain cell processes but, most amazing of all, had actually increased the number of synapses, the contact points through which brain cells communicate with each other.

Another recent study indicates that these changes in brain structure correlate with improved brain function. A 6-month program of exercise improved the memories of a group of older adults, resulting in their faster and more accurate performance on memory tasks. Scanning images showed brain activity patterns in these older individuals' brains to be similar to those seen in young brains. But why would exercising the body improve the mind?

Numerous studies have shown that adults who lose substantial muscle or bone mass increase their risk of developing dementia (including Alzheimer's disease) as they age. Likewise, studies have repeatedly shown that exercise, particularly resistance exercise, such as weight lifting, helps offset the gradual loss of muscle and bone mass that occurs in us all as the years go by. Building lean body mass requires a coordinated interplay of a number of growth factors, released in response to exercise, in a nutritionally enriched body—that is, one that has all the necessary raw materials the body will require to build muscle and/or bone. It's easy to see how running or lifting weights can strengthen the muscles in the legs or arms and cause them to grow. However, it's not so clear how they would affect the brain. But although the connection between exercise and strengthening the brain is far less obvious, it is no less important. The same sort of interplay between growth factor release and a rich supply of raw material building blocks occurs in the brain as well.

Research done in both laboratory animals and humans has shown that exercise increases the amounts of specific brain factors that stimulate growth and repair, especially in the memory centers. One such factor is brain-derived neurotrophic factor (BDNF), which helps boost the formation of a richer network of interconnections among brain cells. These communication channels are vital for learning and memory. BDNF also encourages the growth of new brain cells and protects existing brain cells from the damage related to chronic stress and lack of sleep.

Both aerobic activities (walking, swimming, rowing, biking) and resistance exercise (weight lifting and, to some extent, Pilates) have proven valuable in raising BDNF levels, suggesting that any sort of physical activity is good for brain building. Because BDNF helps the brain form new connections and keep older ones in good repair, it behooves us all—if we hope to maintain our faculties—to keep levels of this brain growth stimulator high and give it plenty of circuitry to work on. Let's take a look at how best to do this.

Cross-Train Your Brain

As noted, the brain works by building a complex network of interconnections among brain cells as we experience new things. From before birth until we trundle off this mortal plane, each new thing we learn, experience, see, hear, feel, say, or do hooks up a new circuit. Repetition solidifies the circuits we build, but they weaken or disconnect entirely with disuse or neglect. The phrase "Use it or lose it!" is nowhere truer than in keeping a keen edge on your mental abilities. That's why I recommend not only that you exercise but that you engage in a wide and often-changing pattern of activity. Although your heart and lungs may benefit if you simply choose to walk or bike each day, and although those (or any) activities will keep some portions of your circuitry dusted off and working well, it's important to challenge yourself in new ways, physically and mentally, so as not to let other circuits rust.

Don't get stuck in an exercise rut; change up your routine. Select a number of activities you enjoy—perhaps walking, swimming, weight training, and yoga—and rotate your workout schedule among them. Then, in addition to what you generally do for exercise, pick up something entirely new or something you haven't done in a while; ride a bike or foot-propelled scooter; try Pilates; learn ballroom dancing, square dancing, or tai chi; or take up golf, softball, Ping-Pong, or tennis to challenge hand–eye coordination and refine your reflexes. Activities such as dancing, tai chi, and yoga that involve learning new and ever more complicated patterns engage both mind and body and are especially good ones. Give whatever new activity that appeals to you a try.

If you have children or grandchildren, don't just watch them play; play with them. Simply keeping up with their pace can be a good workout, but the games kids love to play often require bending, hopping, skipping, and balancing plus innovation, imagination, and quick reactions—all activities that engage different portions of the brain from what you may regularly use and hence light up neglected brain circuits. After all, what could be better for keeping a brain (or a body) young than doing the activities that kids do to form and solidify the connections to begin with?

SAVE YOUR BRAIN

Living an active life will help keep your brain young and your reflexes sharp, but it does come with one caution: If you know from the assessment in Chapter 3 that you are at higher risk for developing memory problems, I would recommend that you not engage in activities that carry a high risk of head trauma.

Activities such as boxing, football, and soccer, which entail a high likelihood of taking repeated blows to the head, can increase your risk for memory loss; that connection is pretty obvious. But remember the research suggesting that perhaps jogging can put you at risk, too. Because the brain floats in a cushioning layer of fluid, pounding the pavement mile after mile, day after day, year in and year out bounces the brain up against the skull, which may be as harmful as the direct, repeated blows a boxer takes to the head. So, if your personal or family history puts you at high risk for memory loss with age, your brain might be better served if you stick to brain-saving activities, such as walking, dancing, swimming, biking, rowing, and the like to keep yourself aerobically fit. And don't forget weight training, which is the best activity of all for releasing BDNF.

MENTAL TRAINING

Ever wish you could make something happen just by thinking it? At one time or another we probably all have wished we could, but believe it or not, when it comes to improving brain function, your wish may come true. Exciting new research has revealed that we can literally think ourselves smarter; just using the brain actually increases the number of connections among brain cells. The more we think, the better our brains function—and here's a welcome surprise—at any age. In fact, older brains may have an advantage.

The kind of memory loss that first begins to afflict people as they age affects what are referred to as the brain's *executive functions* (see Chapter 2), which are housed in its frontal lobes. They involve such things as planning, decision making, flexible thinking, deductive reasoning, and working memory. Working memory requires the capacity to juggle several mental balls at once and to remember what you've done before and what you need to do next. It is what allows us to "hold that thought." These skills are among the most sophisticated of the brain's capabilities and among the most time intensive to acquire, in large measure because they come least naturally to us. We spend the better portion of our youth developing them, but, unfortunately, if we don't use them often *and in novel ways*, they're among the first mental abilities we lose later in life. As we age, we tend to become facile with the skills we use frequently and depend on day to day in our work or habitual leisure activities to the detriment of others we use less often. The good news, however, is that these high-level functions, the first to recede from disuse, respond strikingly well to retraining.

Getting a rusty brain back on track requires time and effort for sure, but the payback is well worth it. Think about how hard it was for you to learn to ride a bike. After suffering through scraped knees and banged elbows, you were soon jumping curbs, weaving between potholes, and riding with no hands. The skills you acquired became second nature for you; your brain seemed to perform them without any conscious thought on your part. If you haven't ridden a bike in a while, try it. I guarantee you will be uncomfortable at first, even surprised at how difficult riding a bike can be. But with practice, very soon you'll be comfortably gliding down the road again.

Remembering is no different. Young brains recall facts quickly; with age, however, the ability to call up information quickly on demand—simple things, from where you put your keys or reading glasses to where you parked the car—becomes increasingly tougher. And stammering with a blank look on your face, unable to recall the name of an important client at a social function can be not only embarrassing but potentially costly. Remembering is a skill that involves retrieving particular bits of information from storage, and it requires the brain's executive functions for guidance on where it was within the brain that we tucked each tidbit away. If the rich brain cell to brain cell connections in the frontal lobes begin to falter from disuse, the ability to quickly find the needed bits of information fails.

Just like learning to ride a bike again, you must consciously retrain your brain to do some of the things that at one time came easily. With committed practice, you can dust off the rusty connections and reward yourself with better mental clarity, improved memory, sharper focus, increased attention, and quicker reaction speed. You'll learn how to do it in this chapter.

WORKING ON RECALL

Researchers test brain function in a variety of ways, one of which is the ability to recall recently learned information. On tests of short-term recall, younger people almost universally outperform older ones. The tests often require the subject to memorize a list of neutral items—meaning random items without any type of special attachment or relevance—and recalling them after a time. The neutrality of the items is key in putting all subjects on equal footing, because we much more easily remember information that is unusual, meaningful to us, or to which emotion or some special significance is attached. For instance, if you drive a Ford and you were asked to remember a list of types of cars that included Ford, remembering that brand would be a snap. Or if in history class you were asked to remember what year the Battle of Hastings took place and you were born in October of 1966, it would be much easier for you to remember the date: 1066. The number combination would have special significance to you.

To remember something, particularly as we grow older, it helps to *make* it unforgettable by attaching it to something meaningful to make it stand out. Attaching a memory to something meaningful engages the executive centers in the frontal lobe of your brain and makes them work. Just as with relearning how to ride a bike, practice makes perfect; regularly engaging in memorization and problem-solving based on this attaching significance approach can actually shake the cobwebs from that dusty frontal lobe, make your brain more agile, and improve your memory recall.

THE BTP METHOD

I have devised a simple three-step memory system within the Brain Trust Program based on this approach; I call it the BTP method, standing not for Brain Trust Program, as you might first think, but for Behold, Train, and Prompt. It's quick, easy, and surprisingly effective; and best of all, it doesn't require listening to CDs or watching videos to become adept at using it. With it you can rapidly and easily improve your memory skills by developing a better filing and retrieval system for the things you need to remember.

Step One: Behold

According to various dictionary definitions, the word *behold* means to perceive to the fullest extent; to understand; to gain perspective about; to investigate, observe, absorb, comprehend, or assimilate every detail of. To behold something requires more than just taking a cursory glance; it can't be done with distractions to your attention. To behold something, anything, takes time and dedication and effort. It's active, not passive. Let me illustrate the difference.

Imagine yourself going somewhere in an unfamiliar city as the passenger in a car. The car stops at stop signs, turns at intersections, obeys traffic lights, one-way street signs, traverses on-ramps and off-ramps, and winds through roundabouts as you travel through neighborhoods you don't know, until you finally arrive safely at your destination. If you were asked to drive that route again, alone, the next day you would probably find it difficult, perhaps even impossible. Why? Because you were just along for the ride; the driver had things under control and required no input from you. He or she chose the route, followed the rules of the road, negotiated the lights, turns, and exits and was the active participant in the trip; if asked to, the driver could probably have pretty easily followed the same route again. You, the passenger, however, were just a passive observer. If brain researchers could have scanned each of your brains during this trip, the driver's frontal lobe circuits would have been lit up like a Christmas tree and yours would have been relatively quiet. Activating the executive functions in the frontal lobe results in better memory recall.

One secret to cultivating a sharper memory is to train yourself to pay attention to details, to become a world-class observer or, in other words, to be the driver. The details of something make it stand out and make recalling it easier; the more of your senses you can engage in the process, the more active your brain's executive centers will become and the sharper your memory will be.

The Detective Game

An easy way to begin this training process is to pretend you are a detective at a crime scene and that it's imperative that you take in and remember even the tiniest, most trivial detail to solve the crime. Start by sitting in a chair in a quiet room—your pretend crime scene. Look around the room for a moment and then close your eyes. Ask yourself to describe the room. What color are the walls? Is there a window? On which wall? Does it have a shade? Is it open or shut? What kind of floor does the room have? Are there rugs? Where? What furniture is present in the room? What color is the sofa or chair? Is there a table? Where? A lamp? Is it on or off? What color is its shade? What shape? Are there pictures on the wall? Of what? Is there other artwork present? What kind? Where is it in the room?

Open your eyes and check yourself. You'll be amazed at how little you actually saw as you surveyed your surroundings. Now repeat the exercise, but start by following these general guidelines:

- Look at the room from a global perspective; notice its general layout, including furniture arrangement; rug location; wall, window, and door locations; wall hangings; large pictures; and general architectural details, such as built-in bookshelves, fireplace, entertainment center, and cabinetry. Then take in the smaller elements of decoration, such as books, figurines, photos, lamps, and knickknacks.

- Next, divide the room into quadrants and examine how each of the four parts is arranged and how the four parts come together to make the whole room.

- Now focus on specific items and note each one in as much detail as possible. For instance, if there is a fireplace, what shape is it? Does it have a glass door or a screen? Is the trim brass, silver, black? What about the grate? What is it made of? Is there wood in the fire box? How much? Is there a hearth? What is it made of? Is there a mantle? What is it made of? And so on. Include as much detail as you can. Refer to colors not simply as red or blue, but force yourself to be specific about the shade of color. Is it the blue-green of aquamarine? The blue-violet of periwinkle? The deep almost black-blue of cobalt or navy? The blue of a robin's egg or the sky? Comment on the textures in the room, both how they look and how they feel. Force yourself to use highly descriptive adjectives; if a surface is rough, is it crackly like parchment, grainy, gnarled, or nubby? Create the most vivid picture you can, one that evokes sights, sounds, aromas, textures, and colors. Together, these details will create for you a memorable image and a memorable image leaves a stronger and more lasting memory trace; it etches itself more deeply in the circuitry of your brain.

You can use the same detective technique to enhance your recall in almost any area, from what you had for dinner last night to the theme of a movie or the plot of a novel to the names of people you meet at a party or the list of items you need to pick up from the store. The next time you are at a party, try this technique with someone you've never met. Start from across the room (so you aren't so conspicuous) by noticing the contours of the person's face; his eyebrows, ears, nose, slope of the jaw or forehead; his general build; and his hair color and style. Is there something particularly interesting or unique that stands out to you? Once you've made your long-distance observations, introduce yourself to the person and strike up a conversation. Is there anything unusual or of significance to you about the person's first or last name, what he does for a living, where he is from? For instance, say it's a gentleman with a square jaw like Robert Redford's and the man happens to be named Mr. Roberts. Once you've planted the memory with a hook like that, you'll likely not forget his name when you see his face in the future. You've added meaning to this new memory by attaching it to something already solidly in your memory files and made accessing this tidbit of information, the gentleman's name, much easier.

Step Two: Train

Just as with learning (or relearning) any skill, practice makes perfect; whether it's learning to recite a poem, play a piano piece from memory, or juggle, repetition is the key to etching a memory deeply and making its retrieval effortless. I learned the power of repetition when I was in medical school, struggling my way through a course in physiology. I began by trying to read entire chapters, plowing through page after page, trying to understand and file away as much as I could of the mountain of information I had to cover. When I finished a chapter, however, I realized that although I'd read it all, I really hadn't learned much of it. I realized then that somehow, despite the time I had invested, my brain had been simply along for the ride (like a passenger in the car) and hadn't been engaged actively in the learning process.

I decided to change my approach to one much more like the detective training method. I would read a page and then stop, cover the book, close my eyes, and review mentally what I'd read on that page from top to bottom in as much detail as possible, often saying it aloud. I noticed that repeating the information out loud seemed to make it stick even better, which makes sense since it stimulates both speech and hearing pathways in the brain.

Next, I would quickly scan the page to fill in anything I'd left out the first time, which took no more than 10 or 15 seconds but forced me to go over the material in a slightly different fashion a third time. Through purposeful repetition, you can train your brain effectively. It is interesting that just knowing that I was going to be tested (albeit self-tested) helped me more sharply focus my attention on the material during my first read through; it made me a better observer of details in the behold part of the scheme.

I discovered this triple *R* training process (read-recall-review) to be quite effective in helping me learn, and it vastly improved my ability to remember what I'd read. I've recommended read-recall-review countless times to my school- and college-aged patients, family members, and friends; but lest you think it applies only to those in the formal educational system, consider this: How often do you find yourself, when reading for work or pleasure, having to reread paragraphs countless times? When that happens, your brain isn't engaging fully in the process, you're spinning your wheels and wasting your time, because you will not remember the information. Employ the triple *R* method, even if you're just reading an article in the newspaper. Read the paragraph, close your eyes, and attempt to recall the important points— aloud if possible. Then review the paragraph and see what, if anything, you missed. Go on to the next paragraph and do the same. Before long, you'll notice that when you read, your brain automatically engages more effectively.

Step Three: Prompt

Sometimes, all it takes to remember something easily, perhaps a list of all the items you need to pick up from the store, is to hook the items to something already memorable or familiar or to connect them in an unusual way that will prompt your memory. For example, let's say you needed to collect these items for a scavenger hunt for your daughter's birthday party: a watermelon, finger paints, a pair of socks, a 10-penny nail, a softball, and a video of *The Little Mermaid*. Without reviewing them, close your eyes and try to repeat the list. Were you able to do it? Do you think you would still remember it when you got to the store, or more likely, several stores? If not, you could certainly simply write out the list, but that wouldn't further your goal of improving your memory and keeping the memory circuits free of cobwebs and rust. Instead, try building a picture that includes all the elements on your list—the more bizarre the better. Envision this picture: the Little Mermaid, wearing hot pink socks on her tail fins, standing on a watermelon, painting a picture of a softball with a 10-penny nail driven through the middle of it. Now close your eyes and repeat the list. Were you able to remember all six items? Try again in half an hour and I'll bet you'll be able to remember them. I still remember lists I learned more than 25 years ago using techniques like this one.

In medical school, students are expected to learn an astounding number of facts. In gross anatomy, our instructors told us we would learn approximately 8,000 new terms—the name of every muscle, ligament, and tendon; every bump on every bone; every nerve and artery, where each goes and what it supplies; every gland and who discovered it, and on and on and on. You reach a point somewhere in those first years, when you think if the instructors expect you to learn one more fact you're surely going to have to boot another one out to make room in your brain. To keep it all straight, we relied on memory joggers, called mnemonics—nonsense words, phrases, or nursery-like rhymes attached usually to the first letters of the items we needed to remember. Entire booklets have been written cataloging the many memory joggers medical students the world over have come up with to prompt their recall of endless lists of names and facts they must commit to memory. For instance, remembering the names of the eight bones of the wrist—the scaphoid, lunate, triquetral, pisiform, trapezium, trapezoid, capitate, and hamate—is easier if you remember, instead: "Some lovers try positions that they can't handle" or "Tom Thumb can heave passes to Lake Superior."

If it works better for you, use the nonsense mnemonic technique instead of the bizarre picture method to help you remember. For example, to re-member all the items you needed to gather for your daughter's party, try a mnemonic, such as "Will Fido sniff Nell's bass violin?" It's easier to remember this nonsensical sentence than the list, but the sentence will jog your memory for watermelon, finger paint, socks, nail, ball, and video. Or how about the stops you need to make to gather the items? You'll need to go to the grocery store, art store, department store, hardware store, sporting goods store, and video rental store. Try reciting that list cold. Now, make a non-sense word mnemonic with the first letters of each stop: GADHSV. Reciting the letters aloud, they sort of have a natural rhythm and rhyme that will make it memorable, even though it's nonsensical. But what about flipping the last three around and adding words: Get A Daughter's VHS? Now you've made a connection that's sure to lodge in your head, since VHS is a familiar se-quence of letters and it and video store are already closely linked in your brain. Now can you remember the stops easily?

Doing these simple exercises regularly will help improve your recall and you'll find yourself almost instantly devising clever, funny, or unusual mem-ory joggers when you need to be able to remember a list of items. In the brain, it's use it or lose it; engaging your brain in memory tasks will keep those connections open and the circuitry polished. Make it a habit.

The Business of Leisure

Leisure time is for fun and relaxation; but as you'll soon see, it's also serious business for those of us who want to keep our brains ticking. It may seem counterintuitive that having fun and not working can actually be good for the brain, but numerous studies since the mid-1990s suggest that this is so. Moreover, the research indicates that our daily behaviors can even alter the cellular structure of our brain. For instance, when adult rats are housed in complex environments containing mirrors, balls, and other toys they can play with or manipulate, their brains actually look different under the microscope than those of their rat friends housed in more Spartan surroundings.

The brain cells of the enriched-environment rats had longer and more complex dendrites—the cells' signal-receiving projections, sort of like antennae—and more cell to cell connection sites, all of which make the brain a more powerful computer. Tests in infant humans, based on function rather than architecture, bear this out; children raised in an enriched and stimulating environment perform better on tests than those raised in bare surroundings. But even old brains respond to stimulation. Elderly rodents living in complex environments show improved performance on learning, memory, and motor performance tests, such as maze running, just as their younger kin. Exactly what happens to cause this improvement isn't clearly understood, but it appears to involve the interplay among brain chemicals that enhance nerve cell growth and repair, certain hormones, and the signaling chemicals (neurotransmitters) that allow the brain cells to communicate with each other. That's well and good for rats, but does it apply to us?

Emerging data suggest that it does; that what we do, enjoy, and surround ourselves with (our enriched or complex environment, if you will) throughout our lives can have a major influence on how gracefully our brains age. Some scientists feel that at least part of the explanation involves a concept called *neural reserve*, which you can think of as the brain's reserve capacity, sort of a mental savings account of spare gray and white matter that we build in response to interaction with our environment as we grow and develop.

The brain, given the needed stimulation and opportunity, builds a significant amount of redundancy into its interconnections—that is, it wires many alternate routes to perform any particular mental task. That way, if one route is knocked out by trauma or disease, other routes are in place to take up the slack. These redundant connections are your reserve pool to draw from, if needed; and the more of them you build, the better off you are. From a functional standpoint, the bigger the neural savings account you've built, the more brain cells you can afford to lose and still maintain good mental performance. So how do you go about building your reserve fund? You do it by learning and by continually challenging your brain in new ways throughout your life. In childhood this builds a better brain, and in adulthood this helps maintain it.

Science has documented the fact that the more years of formal education a person has, the greater his or her neural reserve. Followed over time, these more-educated individuals seem to function better and experience less loss of mental horsepower. But education comes in many forms and continues (or should, if keeping the brain sharp is the goal) long after the cap and gown have been packed away. Clinical research supports this link between ongoing mental stimulation—including not only formal learning but the diversity, novelty, and frequency of participation in mentally stimulating leisure-time activities—and the preservation of neural reserve.

One very interesting study, called the Bronx Aging Study, followed more than 400 people (age 75 and older and still mentally sharp) for a period of more than 5 years. At the beginning of the study, researchers compiled data about the subjects' frequency of participation in such brain-stimulating activities as reading, writing, working crossword puzzles, playing board or card games, engaging in group discussions, or playing music to generate what the scientists termed a cognitive activity score. Each 1-point increase in this composite score predicted a 5 percent decrease in an invidual's risk for developing significant memory loss. The findings of that study correlate well with another aging study that included more than 5,000 residents over age 55 in an urban Chinese community. The second study, also based on frequency of participation in similar mentally stimulating activities, showed the same 5 percent fall in risk for memory impairment for every 1-point increase in an invidual's composite score; and these beneficial results came mainly from reading and from playing traditional Chinese board games such as mahjong. In an interesting side note, however, researchers also found a 20 percent increased risk of subsequent mental decline associated with watching television, once again pointing out the importance of engaging the brain actively versus just letting it go along for the ride.

Participation in new, challenging, mentally stimulating leisure activities not only in the second half of your life but throughout your lifetime has a proven track record in keeping your brain keen. Opting for the kinds of leisure activities that provide a complex and enriched mental environment—reading, writing, playing an instrument, working puzzles, playing card or board games, participating in discussion groups, taking adult education classes—will help you build and maintain the best brain you can. And the best functioning brain is also the one that will most effectively resist the ravages of time.

To get you started and dust off those rusty brains, I have devised a set of training exercises. I think of them much like a total gym for the brain. They consist of a series of daily mental workouts. I've included a brain testing regimen that you should use to assess your progress. It consists of two tests, each of which is to be taken on the same day once every 4 weeks. Think of these tests much like you would view midterm quizzes when you were in school. Teachers devise such tests to assess your proficiency in the subject matter. Graphs are provided so you can plot your scores on both the training and testing components of the Brain Trust Program exercises. *Before* getting started on the training program, take the two baseline (Week 0) tests on pages 170 and 176 to establish your present level of performance, and plot your scores for each on the appropriate graphs.

Mental Gymnastics

The mental gymnastics part of the Brain Trust Program comprises 28 sets of seemingly simple calculations (exercises) and two brain function tests, the Memory Function Test and the Trail Making Test. The exercises are designed to work out many regions of the brain simultaneously. The two tests give you a way to track your progress.

In the arena of physical fitness, it has been demonstrated repeatedly that maximal gains in muscle mass are achieved only when weight-training exercises are performed properly. The same logic applies to the brain. To optimize functional improvements, the directions given here must be followed *exactly as described*. It might be helpful to take a moment and discuss the reasons for this. The directions follow from observations of humans whose brains were studied while they were performing specific mental tasks.

The mental tasks were formulated so they could be performed while in a brain-scanning device called an MRI scanner. A specialized imaging protocol was used that allowed the researchers to identify which areas of the brain were activated during the performance of the task. This is called functional MRI (fMRI) scanning. The word *functional* was chosen to describe this type of scan because it refers to the fact that certain regions of the brain are activated to perform the specific function being called for.

Just as activating more muscle fibers allows for greater power generation, activating more regions of the brain allows for enhanced brain computational ability. Tasks that cause more of the surface of the brain to light up on the fMRI scan also correlate with enhanced performance, better recall, and improved learning. What this means is that mental exercises that turn on more of the brain translate into better learning. Hence I have chosen exercises that require input from the greatest number of nerve cells. They consist of a series of timed sequential arithmetic calculations that must be read aloud as they are performed and the result written out in words. The detailed directions follow.

How could such seemingly simple arithmetic calculations stimulate so much of the brain? Let's walk through the sample calculation: $9 - 5 + 3 =$ _____. The brain must first focus on step one: nine minus five, which equals four. Then, while still holding this result in your memory banks, the next calculation must be performed: four plus three equals seven. However, instead of writing the number 7 in the appropriate space on the answer sheet, the word *seven* must be written. This forces your brain to translate the figure 7 into the word *seven*. Not only is it necessary to perform the calculations, you must also say each of them out loud: nine minus five equals four plus three equals seven. This verbalizing adds yet another step of complexity. Such a process calls on language skills as well as calculation skills, and the need to flip-flop back and forth from one to the other. It activates the brain centers responsible for the arithmetic calculation part of the task, and then sends a message to the language centers so you can think of the words and then ultimately to the motor regions that translate the thought into the production of speech. Because the entire exercise is timed, this adds additional brain-processing demands. If we were able to visualize which parts of the brain such processing requirements call on, we would see that almost all of the brain is required.

The following brain functions are necessary for completion of the Mental Gymnastics Training exercises if they are performed exactly as prescribed: working memory, calculation, language, focus, attention, hand–eye coordination, visual processing, auditory processing, mental-processing speed, motor (movement) function, tactile (touch) processing, spatial processing, vigilance, mental flexibility, and communication between both halves of the brain, to name just a few.

Note: These exercises are designed to be used for your personal benefit and not as a competition among family or friends.

MENTAL GYMNASTICS TRAINING

As a reminder, before you begin the exercises complete the baseline (Week 0) versions of the Memory Function Test (page 170) and the Trail Making Test (page 176) and plot your results on the appropriate graph.

Complete one page of training exercises, consisting of 40 calculations, each day for 28 days. You should check your results for accuracy (see pages 166–169 for the correct answers) and plot your daily results on the Mental Gymnastics Performance Record on page 165.

At the end of the first 28-day round of exercises (sometime on day 28 after the last training session), you should complete the Memory Function Test and the Trail Making Test for week 4 and record your results.

On the following day, you are to start the next 28-day cycle of Brain Training exercises followed by the Memory Function Test and Trail Making Test for week 8. This process is to be repeated every 4 weeks.

To exercise your brain you will need a quiet room, a pencil, a piece of lined paper, and a stopwatch or timer. At the top of the page, record the day (Day 1, Day 2, and so on) and date. Write the numbers 1 through 40 on your lined paper. You will record your answers to each of the 40 calculations next to the respective number on the paper.

- Read each calculation *out loud* as you work through each step of the calculation. For example, "three times two equals six, minus four equals." All calculations must be done in your head. Do not use the pencil to write out the calculations first and then transfer them to the lined sheet.

- On your lined paper, *write out* the answer to each calculation next to its number, 1 through 40. *Note:* The answer must be written out in words. For example, *four* or *nine* not *4* or *9*. Proceed as rapidly as you can reliably accomplish the arithmetic calculations. If you write down more than one or two incorrect answers you need to slow down to improve your accuracy. (An answer key is provided on pages 166–169.)

- When you are finished, write down the time, in seconds, that it takes to complete all 40 calculations. Record the time on the Mental Gymnastics Performance Record on page 165. The graph provides space to mark 28 test results. Photocopy this graph so that you can use it for subsequent exercise rounds. Check your answers against the answer key. You may want to adjust your speed to increase accuracy in subsequent exercises.

- At the end of each cycle of 28 exercises, complete the corresponding Memory Function Test and the Trail Making Test for that 4-week cycle. These are both to be completed on day 28 sometime after you have finished the Mental Gymnastics session. Record your score for each on pages 174 and 191, respectively.

MENTAL GYMNASTICS EXERCISE

Day 1   Date_____   Time_____

1. $3 \times 4 - 5 =$ _____   11. $8 - 5 \times 2 =$ _____   21. $6 + 2 \times 1 =$ _____   31. $9 - 7 \times 3 =$ _____

2. $7 - 3 + 6 =$ _____   12. $3 \times 5 - 8 =$ _____   22. $4 - 1 \times 3 =$ _____   32. $7 + 4 - 3 =$ _____

3. $2 + 4 - 1 =$ _____   13. $6 - 4 \times 3 =$ _____   23. $1 + 7 \times 1 =$ _____   33. $9 - 7 - 1 =$ _____

4. $8 + 3 - 2 =$ _____   14. $5 - 2 + 7 =$ _____   24. $3 \times 4 - 7 =$ _____   34. $8 - 5 \times 2 =$ _____

5. $1 + 4 + 4 =$ _____   15. $2 + 8 - 5 =$ _____   25. $2 \times 5 - 3 =$ _____   35. $7 \times 2 - 5 =$ _____

6. $4 \times 4 - 7 =$ _____   16. $3 - 1 \times 4 =$ _____   26. $4 \times 3 - 5 =$ _____   36. $2 \times 5 - 3 =$ _____

7. $5 - 4 + 8 =$ _____   17. $9 + 4 - 3 =$ _____   27. $4 \times 2 - 4 =$ _____   37. $1 + 6 - 2 =$ _____

8. $9 - 4 \times 2 =$ _____   18. $7 - 1 + 3 =$ _____   28. $8 - 1 + 3 =$ _____   38. $4 - 1 \times 3 =$ _____

9. $6 \times 3 - 9 =$ _____   19. $3 + 6 - 5 =$ _____   29. $1 \times 8 - 5 =$ _____   39. $3 + 5 - 7 =$ _____

10. $3 + 8 - 5 =$ _____   20. $7 - 1 + 4 =$ _____   30. $5 \times 3 - 7 =$ _____   40. $6 - 3 + 7 =$ _____

Day 2   Date_____   Time_____

1. $4 \times 3 - 5 =$ _____   11. $6 \times 2 - 5 =$ _____   21. $4 \times 4 - 8 =$ _____   31. $1 + 6 - 4 =$ _____

2. $3 \times 4 - 5 =$ _____   12. $3 - 1 + 8 =$ _____   22. $2 \times 9 - 8 =$ _____   32. $3 \times 4 - 7 =$ _____

3. $9 - 3 + 2 =$ _____   13. $2 + 6 \times 1 =$ _____   23. $1 + 7 - 5 =$ _____   33. $2 \times 6 - 4 =$ _____

4. $3 + 8 - 4 =$ _____   14. $8 + 7 - 9 -$ _____   24. $9 - 7 + 8 =$ _____   34. $7 \times 2 - 5 =$ _____

5. $8 \times 2 - 6 =$ _____   15. $7 \times 2 - 8 =$ _____   25. $2 \times 9 - 8 =$ _____   35. $5 - 2 \times 2 =$ _____

6. $7 + 2 - 3 =$ _____   16. $8 + 3 - 5 =$ _____   26. $2 \times 8 - 7 =$ _____   36. $7 - 6 \times 6 =$ _____

7. $1 + 3 \times 2 =$ _____   17. $9 - 4 + 3 -$ _____   27. $2 + 6 + 2 =$ _____   37. $7 \times 2 - 4 -$ _____

8. $2 + 6 - 1 =$ _____   18. $4 + 6 - 3 -$ _____   28. $6 \times 3 - 9 =$ _____   38. $4 - 2 \times 4 =$ _____

9. $7 + 2 - 8 =$ _____   19. $6 + 8 - 5 =$ _____   29. $7 + 1 - 6 =$ _____   39. $8 + 4 - 7 =$ _____

10. $2 \times 6 - 8 =$ _____   20. $5 + 6 - 7 =$ _____   30. $2 \times 4 - 3 =$ _____   40. $3 \times 2 - 4 =$ _____

Day 3   Date_____   Time_____

1. $7+8-6=$_____   11. $4+7-5=$_____   21. $6\times2-5=$_____   31. $6+4-7=$_____

2. $4-3\times2=$_____   12. $2\times7-4=$_____   22. $5+3\times1=$_____   32. $7\times2-4=$_____

3. $2-1\times9=$_____   13. $9+3-7=$_____   23. $3\times6-8=$_____   33. $4+4-6=$_____

4. $8-5\times3+$_____   14. $7+3-4=$_____   24. $4+6-3=$_____   34. $9-7\times5=$_____

5. $2\times5-3=$_____   15. $1+8-6=$_____   25. $6-4+8=$_____   35. $3\times5-8=$_____

6. $3+6-2=$_____   16. $3+3-5=$_____   26. $2\times8-7=$_____   36. $8+4-7=$_____

7. $1\times7-5=$_____   17. $5\times3-9=$_____   27. $1+3-2=$_____   37. $2\times6-7=$_____

8. $5+6-4=$_____   18. $6+7-4=$_____   28. $9+4-5=$_____   38. $1+6-4=$_____

9. $3\times5-7=$_____   19. $8+6-5=$_____   29. $7+5-6=$_____   39. $4\times4-8=$_____

10. $7-4\times2=$_____   20. $5+3-5=$_____   30. $6+4-2=$_____   40. $3\times2-5=$_____

Day 4   Date _____   Time _____

1. $4+6-2=$ _____   11. $8-5+6=$ _____   21. $5\times2-4=$ _____   31. $6\times2-5=$ _____

2. $6\times2-8=$ _____   12. $9-5\times2=$ _____   22. $4\times3-6=$ _____   32. $6+3-5=$ _____

3. $5+3-7=$ _____   13. $5-4\times7=$ _____   23. $9+5-6=$ _____   33. $3+6-5=$ _____

4. $4\times4-8=$ _____   14. $2\times8-7=$ _____   24. $2+6-7=$ _____   34. $8-4\times2=$ _____

5. $2+7-8=$ _____   15. $7\times2-9=$ _____   25. $3\times6-8=$ _____   35. $2\times4-6=$ _____

6. $7-5\times5=$ _____   16. $3\times5-7=$ _____   26. $1+5+4=$ _____   36. $5-1+4=$ _____

7. $8+8-9=$ _____   17. $2\times8-9=$ _____   27. $8-6+3=$ _____   37. $4\times2+2-$ _____

8. $0-0+5=$ _____   18. $7+2-5=$ _____   28. $0\times3-8=$ _____   38. $9-6\times3=$ _____

9. $3+4-2=$ _____   19. $8-5\times3=$ _____   29. $7-4\times2=$ _____   39. $1+8-6=$ _____

10. $2+5-4=$ _____   20. $8-1-4=$ _____   30. $6+3-7=$ _____   40. $3\times1+6=$ _____

Day 5   Date_____   Time_____

1. $2 \times 7 - 6 =$_____   11. $7 + 3 - 6 =$_____   21. $3 \times 2 - 5 =$_____   31. $1 + 8 - 5 =$_____

2. $5 - 2 \times 2 =$_____   12. $6 + 1 - 2 =$_____   22. $4 + 3 + 2 =$_____   32. $3 - 1 \times 5 =$_____

3. $4 + 5 - 3 =$_____   13. $3 \times 1 + 6 =$_____   23. $2 + 9 - 5 =$_____   33. $8 - 4 + 5 =$_____

4. $9 - 6 \times 2 =$_____   14. $7 - 4 + 3 =$_____   24. $5 + 4 - 5 =$_____   34. $7 - 4 \times 2 =$_____

5. $4 + 3 - 1 =$_____   15. $2 + 6 - 5 =$_____   25. $1 + 5 - 4 =$_____   35. $2 \times 4 - 6 =$_____

6. $1 \times 5 + 3 =$_____   16. $6 - 5 + 4 =$_____   26. $7 - 5 \times 3 =$_____   36. $8 - 6 \times 2 =$_____

7. $9 - 6 \times 3 =$_____   17. $4 \times 4 - 9 =$_____   27. $2 \times 3 + 4 =$_____   37. $9 - 8 + 7 =$_____

8. $3 + 7 - 5 =$_____   18. $1 + 8 - 5 =$_____   28. $9 + 7 - 8 =$_____   38. $2 \times 7 - 5 =$_____

9. $8 \times 2 - 7 =$_____   19. $2 + 6 - 5 =$_____   29. $8 - 5 \times 2 =$_____   39. $4 + 9 - 7 =$_____

10. $9 + 4 - 8 =$_____   20. $5 \times 3 - 7 =$_____   30. $6 - 5 + 7 =$_____   40. $6 + 9 - 7 =$_____

Day 6   Date_____   Time_____

1. $5 \times 3 - 8 =$ _____   11. $4 + 7 - 5 =$ _____   21. $8 - 6 \times 2 =$ _____   31. $7 + 8 - 6 =$ _____

2. $4 + 9 - 5 =$ _____   12. $2 \times 7 - 8 =$ _____   22. $7 + 6 - 9 =$ _____   32. $5 \times 3 - 8 =$ _____

3. $2 \times 4 - 2 =$ _____   13. $3 \times 5 - 6 =$ _____   23. $7 - 2 + 4 =$ _____   33. $2 \times 2 + 5 =$ ____

4. $1 + 7 - 4 =$ _____   14. $6 - 3 \times 2 =$ _____   24. $2 \times 6 - 7 =$ _____   34. $9 + 5 - 7 =$ _____

5. $5 + 7 - 6 =$ _____   15. $1 + 6 - 3 =$ _____   25. $2 \times 5 - 8 =$ _____   35. $4 \times 4 - 8 =$ _____

6. $8 \times 2 - 7 =$ _____   16. $7 \times 2 - 6 =$ _____   26. $1 + 5 - 3 =$ _____   36. $3 \times 4 - 7 =$ _____

7. $2 + 7 - 5 =$ _____   17. $1 + 8 - 3 =$ _____   27. $6 + 7 - 4 =$ _____   37. $7 - 5 + 3 =$ _____

8. $8 + 7 - 9 =$ _____   18. $3 \times 4 - 5 =$ ____   28. $5 - 3 \times 2 =$ _____   38. $8 \times 2 - 7 =$ _____

9. $6 + 8 - 5 =$ _____   19. $9 - 6 \times 2 =$ _____   29. $3 \times 2 - 4 =$ _____   39. $1 + 7 - 5 =$ _____

10. $9 - 6 \times 3 =$ _____   20. $8 + 7 - 6 =$ _____   30. $2 \times 4 + 2 =$ _____   40. $5 \times 3 - 8 =$ _____

Day 7   Date_____   Time_____

1. $4+7-5=$_____   11. $7-5\times3=$_____   21. $8-5\times3=$_____   31. $8+7-9=$_____

2. $6\times2-3=$_____   12. $5-4\times6=$_____   22. $7\times2-6=$_____   32. $9-6\times3=$_____

3. $1+7-5=$_____   13. $2\times4-5=$_____   23. $6-4\times3=$_____   33. $1+6-5=$_____

4. $3\times4-7=$_____   14. $1+9-5=$_____   24. $2\times2+5=$_____   34. $2\times4-2=$_____

5. $5\times3-7=$_____   15. $4\times3-9=$_____   25. $3\times5-8=$_____   35. $5+7-4=$_____

6. $3+7-5=$_____   16. $5+8-7=$_____   26. $9+7-8=$_____   36. $4\times3-8=$_____

7. $8+5-7=$_____   17. $4+4+2=$_____   27. $7+7-9=$_____   37. $4\times3-7=$_____

8. $9-6\times3=$_____   18. $6-5+7=$_____   28. $8+5-6=$_____   38. $3\times2+4=$_____

9. $7-2\times2=$_____   19. $9+7-6=$_____   29. $3+8-4=$_____   39. $2\times6-3=$_____

10. $2+5-3=$_____   20. $5-1\times2=$_____   30. $2+9-7=$_____   40. $6\times2-3=$_____

Day 8   Date_____   Time_____

1. $4+7-9=$_____   11. $6-4\times2=$_____   21. $7+5-6=$_____   31. $8\times2-7=$_____

2. $9+3-7=$_____   12. $5\times2-6=$_____   22. $8+5-7=$_____   32. $2\times5-4=$_____

3. $3\times3-4=$_____   13. $2\times4-5=$_____   23. $5\times3-8=$_____   33. $2+3-4=$_____

4. $2\times5-3=$_____   14. $7\times2-9=$_____   24. $6-4\times5=$_____   34. $1+7-5=$_____

5. $8-5\times3=$_____   15. $3+8-7=$_____   25. $2+7-5=$_____   35. $5\times3-7=$_____

6. $9+4-7=$_____   16. $7\times2-8=$_____   26. $6+5-8=$_____   36. $6-2+6=$_____

7. $3\times4-7-$_____   17. $0-1+2=$_____   27. $2+7-5=$___   37. $9\times1-4-$_____

8. $7\times2-6=$_____   18. $3+7-5=$_____   28. $1+7-5=$_____   38. $5\times3-6=$_____

9. $5+7-9=$_____   19. $4+7-5=$_____   29. $3\times2+4=$_____   39. $7-4\times3=$_____

10. $9-7\times5=$_____   20. $2+7-3=$_____   30. $7-3\times2=$_____   40. $6+3-7=$_____

Day 9 Date_____ Time_____

1. $6+7-5=$_____ 11. $5-2\times2=$_____ 21. $2\times7-6=$_____ 31. $3+8-7=$_____

2. $2+6-5=$_____ 12. $3\times4-7=$_____ 22. $6-2+5=$_____ 32. $4-1\times3=$_____

3. $8-4\times2=$_____ 13. $2+7-6=$_____ 23. $3\times2+3=$_____ 33. $2+3-1=$_____

4. $9+6-8=$_____ 14. $8-1+3=$_____ 24. $7+6-9=$_____ 34. $7+6-5=$_____

5. $4\times3-5=$_____ 15. $9-5\times2=$_____ 25. $5\times2-7=$_____ 35. $1+6+2=$_____

6. $7\times2-8=$_____ 16. $2+6-4=$_____ 26. $9-6+7=$_____ 36. $3+9-7=$_____

7. $3\times4-7=$_____ 17. $4\times4-8=$_____ 27. $8-5\times2=$_____ 37. $6\times3-9=$_____

8. $6-1\times2=$_____ 18. $7-5\times5=$_____ 28. $7+1-5=$_____ 38. $9+7-9=$_____

9. $7+6-8=$_____ 19. $3\times5-9=$_____ 29. $2\times4+2=$_____ 39. $8\times2-7=$_____

10. $5+9-7=$_____ 20. $7\times2-8=$_____ 30. $8+7-9=$_____ 40. $6+7-8=$_____

Day 10   Date_____   Time_____

1. $7+6-5=$_____   11. $4\times3-9=$_____   21. $2\times8-7=$_____   31. $7-2\times2=$_____

2. $3+6-4=$_____   12. $4+5-7=$_____   22. $5\times3-5=$_____   32. $9-7+5=$_____

3. $4\times4-8=$_____   13. $9+8-7=$_____   23. $3\times3+1=$_____   33. $8+7-6=$___

4. $2+9-5=$_____   14. $7\times2-9=$_____   24. $8+1-5=$_____   34. $6-4\times3=$_____

5. $6+7-8=$_____   15. $2\times5-6=$_____   25. $4\times3-7=$_____   35. $2+7-6=$_____

6. $8\times2-7=$_____   16. $6\times3-9=$_____   26. $2+7-5=$_____   36. $6+7-9=$_____

7. $5\times3-7=$_____   17. $3\times5-7=$_____   27. $9+3-7=$_____   37. $5+8-6=$_____

8. $2+2\times2=$_____   18. $0+7-5=$_____   28. $5+1-1=$_____   38. $3\times2-4=$_____

9. $7+6-8=$_____   19. $6\times2-5=$_____   29. $2+7+1=$_____   39. $5-1\times2=$_____

10. $9+2-6=$_____   20. $9+4-8=$_____   30. $5\times2-7=$_____   40. $4\times4-9=$_____

Day 11   Date_____   Time_____

1. $4 \times 3 - 7 =$ _____   11. $7 - 4 \times 3 =$ _____   21. $9 - 7 \times 3 =$ _____   31. $8 + 5 - 7 =$ _____

2. $5 + 6 - 4 =$ _____   12. $8 - 6 \times 4 =$ _____   22. $3 \times 4 - 8 =$ _____   32. $9 - 7 + 5 =$ _____

3. $9 - 8 \times 7 =$ _____   13. $3 \times 6 - 9 =$ _____   23. $2 + 8 - 6 =$ _____   33. $4 \times 2 + 2 =$ _____

4. $6 \times 2 - 7 =$ _____   14. $2 \times 7 - 7 =$ _____   24. $7 + 6 - 8 =$ _____   34. $5 \times 1 - 3 =$ _____

5. $2 + 8 - 7 =$ _____   15. $5 + 9 - 7 =$ _____   25. $1 + 6 - 4 =$ _____   35. $3 \times 5 - 8 =$ _____

6. $6 - 5 + 7 =$ _____   16. $4 \times 4 - 9 =$ _____   26. $8 \times 2 - 9 =$ _____   36. $2 + 5 - 3 =$ _____

7. $7 \times 2 - 6 =$ _____   17. $5 \times 2 - 3 =$ _____   27. $6 \times 3 - 8 =$ _____   37. $8 + 7 - 9 =$ _____

8. $3 + 9 - 7 =$ _____   18. $4 + 8 - 6 =$ _____   28. $5 + 1 - 2 =$ _____   38. $2 \times 6 - 7 =$ _____

9. $9 + 5 - 7 =$ _____   19. $8 - 5 \times 2 =$ _____   29. $4 \times 3 - 7 =$ _____   39. $3 \times 5 - 7 =$ _____

10. $6 + 3 - 7 =$ _____   20. $7 + 1 - 6 =$ _____   30. $2 \times 4 - 1 =$ _____   40. $6 - 3 \times 3 =$ _____

Day 12   Date_____ Time_____

1. $7-5+2=$_____   11. $8+6-7=$_____   21. $9+4-8=$_____   31. $2\times5-7=$_____

2. $2+9-6=$_____   12. $2\times8-9=$_____   22. $6+5-7=$_____   32. $5+9-8=$_____

3. $3\times5-7=$_____   13. $6\times1+4=$_____   23. $3\times3+1=$_____   33. $2\times7-8=$_____

4. $6-4\times4=$_____   14. $5+3-2=$_____   24. $7\times2-7=$_____   34. $3+9-6=$_____

5. $5\times3-9=$_____   15. $7+6-5=$_____   25. $2\times5-7=$_____   35. $2\times1+7=$_____

6. $9-5\times2=$_____   16. $1+6-3=$_____   26. $4\times1+6=$_____   36. $3\times4-9=$_____

7. $2\times7-5=$_____   17. $3+7-8=$_____   27. $1+7-5=$_____   37. $8\times2-7=$_____

8. $1+6-4=$_____   18. $4\times3-9=$_____   28. $8-6\times3=$_____   38. $7\times2-9=$_____

9. $4+8-6=$_____   19. $8-7\times3=$_____   29. $5\times1-4=$_____   39. $6\times3-9=$_____

10. $5+7-8=$_____   20. $9+2-8=$_____   30. $6\times2-7=$_____   40. $8-4\times2=$_____

Day 13   Date_____   Time_____

1. $5 \times 3 - 8 =$_____   11. $7 - 5 \times 5 =$_____   21. $8 + 5 - 6 =$_____   31. $2 + 5 - 3 =$_____

2. $7 + 7 - 9 =$_____   12. $3 \times 5 - 9 =$_____   22. $2 + 7 - 5 =$_____   32. $5 - 4 + 9 =$_____

3. $2 \times 2 - 1 =$_____   13. $6 - 5 + 8 =$_____   23. $3 \times 3 + 1 =$_____   33. $7 + 3 - 6 =$_____

4. $3 + 8 - 4 =$_____   14. $2 \times 6 - 5 =$_____   24. $1 + 8 - 3 =$_____   34. $6 + 4 - 7 =$_____

5. $7 - 5 \times 4 =$_____   15. $9 + 3 - 6 =$_____   25. $5 \times 3 - 8 =$_____   35. $3 \times 4 - 9 =$_____

6. $2 + 6 + 1 =$_____   16. $1 \times 6 - 5 =$_____   26. $4 \times 4 - 8 =$_____   36. $2 \times 2 + 6 =$_____

7. $5 - 3 + 7 =$_____   17. $8 + 6 - 7 =$_____   27. $9 - 6 \times 3 =$_____   37. $7 + 6 - 8 =$_____

8. $9 + 2 - 6 =$_____   18. $4 \times 3 - 7 =$_____   28. $6 \times 2 - 7 =$_____   38. $1 + 7 - 5 =$_____

9. $8 - 6 \times 5 =$_____   19. $2 \times 2 + 6 =$_____   29. $3 \times 5 - 8 =$_____   39. $7 + 6 - 7 =$_____

10. $5 + 9 - 7 =$_____   20. $7 - 4 \times 3 =$_____   30. $8 \times 2 - 7 =$_____   40. $2 + 6 - 3 =$_____

Day 14   Date_____   Time_____

1. $9-7+5=$_____   11. $7\times2-6=$_____   21. $8+8-9=$_____   31. $4\times2+2=$_____

2. $5\times3-8=$_____   12. $7-5\times3=$_____   22. $8+3-9=$_____   32. $7+6-8=$_____

3. $4\times3-7=$_____   13. $6+5-7=$_____   23. $5\times2-7=$_____   33. $3\times4-9=$_____

4. $9-7\times2=$_____   14. $3\times5-8=$_____   24. $8-6\times5=$_____   34. $6+5-7=$_____

5. $5+5-6=$_____   15. $2+8-6=$_____   25. $6+8-6=$_____   35. $2+4-5=$_____

6. $2+7-4=$_____   16. $8-5\times3=$_____   26. $1+8+1=$_____   36. $2\times2\times2=$_____

7. $9-8\times5=$_____   17. $2\times5-6=$_____   27. $9-2+3=$_____   37. $5\times3-8=$_____

8. $3\times4-7=$_____   18. $2\times4-5=$_____   28. $5\times2-9=$_____   38. $2\times4+2=$_____

9. $3\times5-7=$_____   19. $1+7-5=$_____   29. $2+9-7=$_____   39. $5-4+8=$_____

10. $7-3\times2=$_____   20. $6+4-3=$_____   30. $3+9-4=$_____   40. $6+5-8=$_____

Day 15   Date_____   Time_____

1. $2+1+7=$_____   11. $7-4\times3=$_____   21. $6+5-7=$_____   31. $9+1-6=$_____

2. $6\times3-9=$_____   12. $7-5\times2=$_____   22. $5\times1+4=$_____   32. $3\times4-7=$_____

3. $1+4\times2=$_____   13. $3\times3+1=$_____   23. $4\times2-6=$_____   33. $6\times2-7=$_____

4. $2\times5-6=$_____   14. $7-5\times5=$_____   24. $3+7-4=$_____   34. $2\times4-1=$_____

5. $5\times3-9=$_____   15. $5-4\times7=$_____   25. $7+5-6=$_____   35. $1+3-2=$_____

6. $7+5-6=$_____   16. $2+6-5=$_____   26. $9-2+3=$_____   36. $7-6+4=$_____

7. $6-5+3=$_____   17. $6\times1+4=$_____   27. $5-3+7=$_____   37. $5-4+7=$_____

8. $7+7-8=$_____   18. $7-6+3=$_____   28. $2+3-1=$_____   38. $3\times2+4=$_____

9. $4\times2-1=$_____   19. $1+7-3=$_____   29. $1\times5+4=$_____   39. $7-5\times5=$_____

10. $3\times3+1=$_____   20. $9-7\times4=$_____   30. $2\times4-7=$_____   40. $6-4\times2=$_____

Day 16   Date_____   Time_____

1. $6 \times 3 - 9 =$ _____

2. $4 - 3 + 6 =$ _____

3. $7 - 2 \times 2 =$ _____

4. $6 + 7 - 4 =$ _____

5. $5 - 3 + 7 =$ _____

6. $1 + 6 + 2 =$ _____

7. $5 + 1 - 4 =$ _____

8. $1 + 1 - 8 =$

9. $2 + 4 - 5 =$ _____

10. $4 \times 2 - 7 =$ _____

11. $6 - 4 \times 4 =$ _____

12. $6 + 1 - 2 =$ _____

13. $8 - 6 \times 5 =$ _____

14. $5 \times 2 - 9 =$ _____

15. $9 + 5 - 6 =$ _____

16. $2 \times 5 - 7 =$ _____

17. $6 - 4 \times 3 =$ _____

18. $5 - 3 \times 1 =$ _____

19. $2 + 1 \times 1 =$ _____

20. $7 - 5 \times 2 =$ _____

21. $6 + 3 - 8 =$ _____

22. $3 \times 5 - 8 =$ _____

23. $7 + 5 - 9 =$ _____

24. $5 \times 2 - 7 =$ _____

25. $7 - 6 + 2 =$ _____

26. $3 \times 5 - 9 =$ _____

27. $1 + 6 - 9 =$ _____

28. $2 \times 2 + 3 =$ _____

29. $7 + 5 - 3 =$ _____

30. $3 \times 1 + 6 =$ _____

31. $2 + 7 + 1 =$ _____

32. $1 \times 5 + 4 =$ _____

33. $2 + 1 + 2 =$ _____

34. $3 + 4 - 6 =$ _____

35. $6 + 4 - 2 -$ _____

36. $3 \times 3 + 1 =$ _____

37. $2 \times 7 - 6 =$ _____

38. $9 - 6 \times 3 =$ _____

39. $9 - 7 \times 3 =$ _____

40. $7 - 4 \times 3 =$ _____

Day 17   Date_____   Time_____

1. $1+9-5=$_____   11. $6\times2-9=$_____   21. $2+8-7=$_____   31. $5+3-7=$_____

2. $3\times5-9=$_____   12. $2+4-5=$_____   22. $7-3\times2=$_____   32. $6-5+4=$_____

3. $5\times2-8=$_____   13. $4\times3-8=$_____   23. $6\times2-5=$_____   33. $7-5\times3=$_____

4. $5\times1+4=$_____   14. $2+9-7=$_____   24. $5\times2-8=$_____   34. $1\times8-7=$_____

5. $9+3-5=$_____   15. $7+6-4=$_____   25. $2\times3+4=$_____   35. $8-7+1=$_____

6. $4\times3-7=$_____   16. $2\times5-6=$_____   26. $7-5\times2=$_____   36. $9+3-5=$_____

7. $5\times2-7=$_____   17. $1+5-3=$_____   27. $7\times2-5=$_____   37. $8+3-6=$_____

8. $2\times6-7=$_____   18. $5+4-7=$_____   28. $7+5-8=$_____   38. $3-2+7=$_____

9. $5\times1+4=$_____   19. $3\times3-1=$_____   29. $6-4\times3=$_____   39. $7-1+2=$_____

10. $6-4\times3=$_____   20. $9+6-8=$_____   30. $4\times3-7=$_____   40. $8+4-5=$_____

Day 18   Date_____   Time_____

1. $7-5\times4=$_____   11. $8-3+5=$_____   21. $2+9-7=$_____   31. $8+5-7=$_____

2. $2+7-9=$_____   12. $1+7-2=$_____   22. $6\times2-7=$_____   32. $3\times3-2=$_____

3. $5\times2-9=$_____   13. $7-5\times4=$_____   23. $7+5-4=$_____   33. $3+1-2=$_____

4. $8+5-7=$_____   14. $4\times2+1=$_____   24. $6\times2-9=$_____   34. $2\times5-7=$_____

5. $5+1+4=$_____   15. $6\times1+2=$_____   25. $7-4\times3=$_____   35. $8+4-5=$_____

6. $5\times3-8=$_____   16. $6\times2-5=$_____   26. $2+7-1=$_____   36. $9-8\times1=$_____

7. $4\times3-7=$_____   17. $3\times3-5=$_____   27. $1+9-5=$_____   37. $8+6-7=$_____

8. $2\times5-7=$_____   18. $8+5-7=$_____   28. $5-4+2=$_____   38. $6+1-5=$_____

9. $4\times3-7=$_____   19. $5+3-6=$_____   29. $8-6\times3=$_____   39. $5\times1+3=$_____

10. $1\times9-5=$_____   20. $6-1+4=$_____   30. $2-1+4=$_____   40. $7-3+4=$_____

Day 19   Date_____   Time_____

1. $8+3-4=$_____   11. $3\times4-7=$_____   21. $5+6-3=$_____   31. $9+1-5=$_____

2. $4\times2+2=$_____   12. $6-4\times5=$_____   22. $9-7+2=$_____   32. $2\times6-8=$_____

3. $3\times3-5=$_____   13. $7-5\times4=$_____   23. $6+6-7=$_____   33. $4\times3-6=$_____

4. $1+7+1=$_____   14. $2+1\times3=$_____   24. $7-5\times4=$_____   34. $5+1-3=$_____

5. $2\times4+1=$_____   15. $7+4-9=$_____   25. $8\times2-7=$_____   35. $6+3-8=$_____

6. $6+7-5=$_____   16. $3\times4-4=$_____   26. $8-6\times5=$_____   36. $8-2-3=$_____

7. $3+7-8=$_____   17. $4+1-2=$_____   27. $7+1-4=$_____   37. $6\times2-5=$_____

8. $4\times2-1=$_____   18. $8+1-5=$_____   28. $7-6\times5=$_____   38. $5\times3-8=$_____

9. $7-5\times4=$_____   19. $9+3-7=$_____   29. $6+3+1=$_____   39. $4+6-8=$_____

10. $9+2-7=$_____   20. $7-5\times4=$_____   30. $8-5\times3=$_____   40. $4\times2+1=$_____

Day 20   Date_____   Time_____

1. $1+7-4=$_____

2. $6-5+4=$_____

3. $6-4\times5=$_____

4. $5-3\times5=$_____

5. $9+2-5=$_____

6. $6+5-7=$_____

7. $4-3+7=$_____

0. $2+4+3=$_____

9. $6+1-3=$_____

10. $6-1\times2=$_____

11. $7-5\times4=$_____

12. $2\times6-7=$_____

13. $4-3\times9=$_____

14. $9-5\times2=$_____

15. $4-2\times5=$_____

16. $7\times2-9=$_____

17. $5-2+3=$_____

18. $6-5+2=$_____

19. $2\times5-7=$_____

20. $8+1-7=$_____

21. $8+5-4=$_____

22. $4\times1+6=$_____

23. $6\times2-9=$_____

24. $6+7-4=$_____

25. $7+4-8=$_____

26. $4+2-5=$_____

27. $7-5+1=$_____

28. $3\times4-5=$_____

29. $4-2\times4=$_____

30. $4+7-3=$_____

31. $9-8+7=$_____

32. $5-3\times3=$_____

33. $2+5-4=$_____

34. $7-5+4=$_____

35. $8-5\times3=$_____

36. $8-5\times3=$_____

37. $5-3\times2=$_____

38. $8+1-5=$_____

39. $8+1-7=$_____

40. $9-7\times3=$_____

Day 21   Date_____   Time_____

1. $5-4\times3=$_____   11. $8+4-7=$_____   21. $7+3-8=$_____   31. $3\times4-8=$_____

2. $6+2-7=$_____   12. $7-5\times4=$_____   22. $6+3-1=$_____   32. $7+2-7=$_____

3. $5\times1+4=$_____   13. $6-4\times2=$_____   23. $8+1-7=$_____   33. $7+4-6=$_____

4. $2\times1+7=$_____   14. $4+5-1=$_____   24. $4-2\times3=$_____   34. $6+1-5=$_____

5. $5-3\times4=$_____   15. $4+1\times2=$_____   25. $3+7-5=$_____   35. $6-5\times7=$_____

6. $1+5-2=$_____   16. $7+1-5=$_____   26. $3\times2+1=$_____   36. $8+3-5=$_____

7. $5-4+7=$_____   17. $3+6-7=$_____   27. $6-4+3=$_____   37. $9+2-7=$_____

8. $4\times4-9=$_____   18. $2\times2+5=$_____   28. $1+5-3=$_____   38. $8-5\times3=$_____

9. $5\times3-8=$_____   19. $7-6+4=$_____   29. $9-6\times2=$_____   39. $7-5\times4=$_____

10. $5+4-3=$_____   20. $2+6-4=$_____   30. $4\times2-1=$_____   40. $3\times4-7=$_____

Day 22   Date_____   Time_____

1. $4-2\times4=$_____   11. $7-1+4=$_____   21. $4+7-6=$_____   31. $7-5\times2=$_____

2. $6-5\times7=$_____   12. $4+2-5=$_____   22. $3\times4-8=$_____   32. $1\times5-4=$_____

3. $3\times3-6=$_____   13. $5-2\times3=$_____   23. $7-4-3=$_____   33. $7+2-6=$_____

4. $5+3-4=$_____   14. $2\times5-8=$_____   24. $4\times3-6=$_____   34. $6+5-9=$_____

5. $5-4+7=$_____   15. $2-1+7=$_____   25. $9+6-8=$_____   35. $4\times2+2=$_____

6. $2\times6-8=$_____   16. $4\times2-5=$_____   26. $9-7\times4=$_____   36. $7+5-9=$_____

7. $2+5-6=$_____   17. $5-1\times2=$_____   27. $6-3\times3=$_____   37. $8-5\times2=$_____

8. $6+1-4=$_____   18. $6+4-7=$_____   28. $2+7-4=$_____   38. $7-6+2=$_____

9. $8-5\times3=$_____   19. $6+1-5=$_____   29. $5-2+7=$_____   39. $7-4\times3=$_____

10. $1+3-2=$_____   20. $2+3-1=$_____   30. $8-6\times4=$_____   40. $5-1\times2=$_____

Day 23   Date_____   Time_____

1. $6-4\times5=$_____   11. $7+1-5=$_____   21. $4-2\times4=$_____   31. $8-2+1=$_____

2. $2+7-3=$_____   12. $5-4\times2=$_____   22. $7-5\times3=$_____   32. $6-5+4=$_____

3. $3\times3-7=$_____   13. $2\times5-7=$_____   23. $4-3+6=$_____   33. $6\times2-9=$_____

4. $7-5\times4=$_____   14. $5-4+2=$_____   24. $2\times4-5=$_____   34. $5-3\times4=$_____

5. $6+1-4=$_____   15. $2\times2-1=$_____   25. $6+1+2=$_____   35. $4\times3-7=$_____

6. $5-3\times5=$_____   16. $3-2+6=$_____   26. $5+1-4=$_____   36. $2\times6-7=$_____

7. $5+4-7=$_____   17. $4-2\times3=$_____   27. $5+2-4=$_____   37. $7-1-2=$_____

8. $6-4+7=$_____   18. $4+1\times2=$_____   28. $6+3-7=$_____   38. $8-5\times3=$_____

9. $6+5-3=$_____   19. $7+2-5=$_____   29. $3+6-8=$_____   39. $8-4+5=$_____

10. $9-5\times2=$_____   20. $5+2-6=$_____   30. $3+1-2=$_____   40. $7+4-5=$_____

Day 24   Date_____   Time_____

1. $5-3\times4=$_____   11. $7+1-5=$_____   21. $4\times2-5=$_____   31. $9+2-5=$_____

2. $4\times3-7=$_____   12. $3\times4-5=$_____   22. $2+7-4=$_____   32. $7-1+3=$_____

3. $5+1-3=$_____   13. $6-2\times2=$_____   23. $7+1-4=$_____   33. $1\times5+3=$_____

4. $5-3\times4=$_____   14. $6+2-4=$_____   24. $4+2-5=$_____   34. $8-7\times5=$_____

5. $4\times2-6=$_____   15. $2+7-5=$_____   25. $7-5+4=$_____   35. $4+6-3=$_____

6. $5-2\times3=$_____   16. $7+3-4=$_____   26. $8+1-6=$_____   36. $6\times2-5=$_____

7. $7-2+3=$_____   17. $8+1-5=$_____   27. $4\times2-7=$_____   37. $6+1-5=$_____

8. $2\times6-0=$_____   18. $5+3-7=$_____   28. $2\times5-3=$_____   38. $7\times2-6=$_____

9. $8-5\times3=$_____   19. $4\times3-7=$_____   29. $2+7-4=$_____   39. $8+5-7=$_____

10. $4\times1+5=$_____   20. $6-4\times3=$_____   30. $8+3-7=$_____   40. $7-3+4=$_____

Day 25   Date_____   Time_____

---

1. $8+1-5=$_____   11. $5+5-8=$_____   21. $2+1+5=$_____   31. $7-2+5=$_____

2. $9+3-5=$_____   12. $8-5\times3=$_____   22. $7+1-3=$_____   32. $7+4-5=$_____

3. $4\times2-7=$_____   13. $7+2-4=$_____   23. $4\times1+2=$_____   33. $7-5\times3=$_____

4. $5+1-2=$_____   14. $6+1-4=$_____   24. $9+3-7=$_____   34. $6-5+4=$_____

5. $7-6+8=$_____   15. $9-7\times5=$_____   25. $4-3+6=$_____   35. $7+2-4=$_____

6. $4\times2+1=$_____   16. $2+6-4=$_____   26. $3+6-2=$_____   36. $4\times3-7=$_____

7. $2+7-5=$_____   17. $6+1-3=$_____   27. $7+1-4=$_____   37. $5\times3-8=$_____

8. $9-6\times3=$_____   18. $3\times4-8=$_____   28. $3+3+3=$_____   38. $7-5\times4=$_____

9. $1+6-5=$_____   19. $3-2\times8=$_____   29. $7+5-4=$_____   39. $1\times7-4=$_____

10. $5\times2-6=$_____   20. $5+2-6=$_____   30. $9+2-4=$_____   40. $3\times4-9=$_____

Day 26   Date_____   Time_____

1. $6-4\times2=$ _____   11. $7+3-4=$ _____   21. $3\times5-8=$ _____   31. $2\times6-7=$ _____

2. $4-1\times3=$ _____   12. $6+1-4=$ _____   22. $4\times2-5=$ _____   32. $5+3-7=$ _____

3. $3+7-9=$ _____   13. $6-3\times3=$ _____   23. $8-5\times3=$ _____   33. $4-3\times6=$ _____

4. $5+2-6=$ _____   14. $4\times2-7=$ _____   24. $6-3\times3=$ _____   34. $2\times2\times2=$ _____

5. $6-5+4=$ _____   15. $7+4-3=$ _____   25. $5-3\times2=$ _____   35. $7+1-3=$ _____

6. $2\times5-7=$ _____   16. $2+7-5=$ _____   26. $5-3\times1=$ _____   36. $8+3-4=$ _____

7. $4-1\times3=$ _____   17. $4+3+1=$ _____   27. $7-1+2=$ _____   37. $5-1+2=$ _____

8. $8+1-6=$ _____   18. $7+2-6=$ _____   28. $4+2-5=$ _____   38. $6+1-4=$ _____

9. $5+1-2=$ _____   19. $7-4\times2=$ _____   29. $8+1-5=$ _____   39. $7-5\times3=$ _____

10. $9+5-4=$ _____   20. $4+3-2=$ _____   30. $8-5\times3=$ _____   40. $7+1-3=$ _____

Day 27   Date_____   Time_____

1. $7-4\times3=$_____   11. $6+1-4=$_____   21. $3\times4-7=$_____   31. $7+1-5=$_____

2. $5+2-6=$_____   12. $3\times5-8=$_____   22. $7+2-1=$_____   32. $3+7-5=$_____

3. $3+5+1=$_____   13. $6-1+4=$_____   23. $4+7-3=$_____   33. $5+1-3=$_____

4. $8+1-4=$_____   14. $7-5\times4=$_____   24. $7+1+2=$_____   34. $2+1\times3=$_____

5. $5-4\times8=$_____   15. $3\times4-9=$_____   25. $6+1-3=$_____   35. $6-2\times2=$_____

6. $5+3-7=$_____   16. $3\times1+6=$_____   26. $3+2-4=$_____   36. $7+2-5=$_____

7. $8-5\times2=$_____   17. $7+2-6=$_____   27. $4\times2+1=$_____   37. $6-3\times2=$_____

8. $9-7+3=$_____   18. $8+5-6=$_____   28. $4+2-5=$_____   38. $3+4-1=$_____

9. $5+3-6=$_____   19. $5-3+4=$_____   29. $7-5\times3=$_____   39. $7+2-5=$_____

10. $7+1-2=$_____   20. $3+6-7=$_____   30. $6+3-4=$_____   40. $5\times2-9=$_____

Day 28   Date_____   Time_____

1. $9+3-5=$_____

2. $5-4+3=$_____

3. $2-1+6=$_____

4. $3\times3-7=$_____

5. $5-3\times4=$_____

6. $2\times2+6=$_____

7. $4-3\times8=$_____

8. $8-5\times3=$_____

9. $6-4\times3=$_____

10. $6+3-5=$_____

11. $6-5\times7=$_____

12. $7+2+1=$_____

13. $5+3-7=$_____

14. $7+1-2=$_____

15. $5+1-4=$_____

16. $6-4\times2=$_____

17. $7+1-6=$_____

10. $7+1-4=$_____

19. $5-1\times2=$_____

20. $6+1-5=$_____

21. $7-5\times4=$_____

22. $7-3+2=$_____

23. $6-4\times3=$_____

24. $8+1-5=$_____

25. $8+1-6=$_____

26. $9+3-7=$_____

27. $6-5+4=$_____

28. $3-1+6=$_____

29. $7-4\times2=$_____

30. $4-2\times2=$_____

31. $3\times2+1=$_____

32. $9-5+2=$_____

33. $5-3\times5=$_____

34. $7+1-4=$_____

35. $5+1-4=$_____

36. $6+1-5=$_____

37. $4\times2+1=$_____

38. $7-4+2=$_____

39. $4-2\times5=$_____

40. $7+1-5=$_____

THE MENTAL GYMNASTICS PERFORMANCE RECORD

Photocopy this graph so you have a fresh copy for each 28-day training period. Record your performance by placing a point on the graph that represents your score (time) for the appropriate training day. Join the daily dots to create a graph of your progress.

Mental Gymnastics Performance Record

Week _____ :

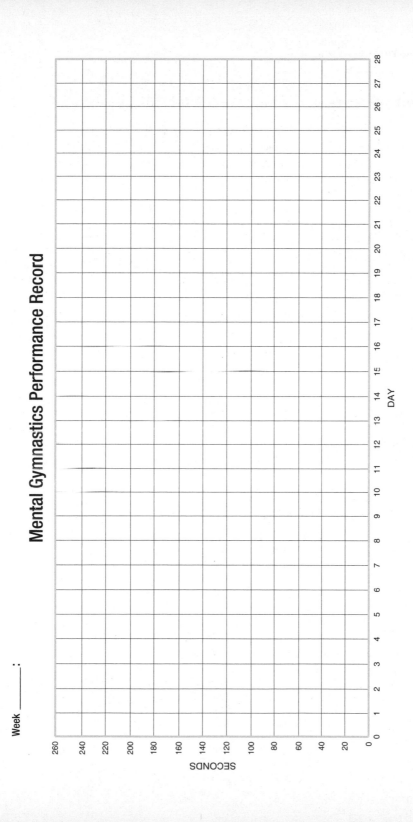

Answer Sheet for Mental Gymnastics Exercises

DAY 1	DAY 2	DAY 3	DAY 4	DAY 5	DAY 6	DAY 7
1. seven	1. seven	1. nine	1. eight	1. eight	1. seven	1. six
2. ten	2. seven	2. two	2. four	2. six	2. eight	2. nine
3. five	3. eight	3. nine	3. one	3. six	3. six	3. three
4. nine	4. seven	4. nine	4. eight	4. six	4. four	4. five
5. nine	5. ten	5. seven	5. one	5. six	5. six	5. eight
6. nine	6. six	6. seven	6. ten	6. eight	6. nine	6. five
7. nine	7. eight	7. two	7. seven	7. nine	7. four	7. six
8. ten	8. four	8. seven	8. ten	8. five	8. six	8. nine
9. nine	9. one	9. eight	9. five	9. nine	9. eight	9. ten
10. six	10. four	10. six	10. three	10. five	10. nine	10. four
11. six	11. seven	11. six	11. nine	11. four	11. six	11. six
12. seven	12. ten	12. ten	12. eight	12. five	12. six	12. six
13. six	13. eight	13. five	13. seven	13. nine	13. nine	13. three
14. ten	14. six	14. six	14. nine	14. six	14. six	14. five
15. five	15. six	15. three	15. five	15. three	15. four	15. three
16. eight	16. six	16. one	16. eight	16. five	16. eight	16. six
17. nine	17. eight	17. six	17. seven	17. seven	17. six	17. ten
18. nine	18. seven	18. nine	18. four	18. four	18. seven	18. eight
19. four	19. nine	19. nine	19. nine	19. three	19. six	19. ten
20. ten	20. four	20. three	20. three	20. eight	20. nine	20. eight
21. eight	21. eight	21. seven	21. six	21. one	21. four	21. nine
22. nine	22. ten	22. eight	22. six	22. nine	22. four	22. eight
23. eight	23. three	23. ten	23. eight	23. six	23. nine	23. six
24. five	24. ten	24. seven	24. one	24. four	24. five	24. nine
25. seven	25. ten	25. ten	25. ten	25. two	25. two	25. seven
26. seven	26. nine	26. nine	26. ten	26. six	26. three	26. eight
27. four	27. ten	27. two	27. five	27. ten	27. nine	27. five
28. ten	28. nine	28. eight	28. ten	28. eight	28. four	28. seven
29. three	29. two	29. six	29. six	29. six	29. two	29. seven
30. eight	30. five	30. eight	30. two	30. eight	30. ten	30. four
31. six	31. three	31. three	31. seven	31. four	31. nine	31. six
32. eight	32. five	32. ten	32. four	32. ten	32. seven	32. nine
33. one	33. eight	33. two	33. four	33. nine	33. nine	33. two
34. six	34. nine	34. ten	34. eight	34. six	34. seven	34. six
35. nine	35. six	35. seven	35. two	35. two	35. eight	35. eight
36. seven	36. six	36. five	36. eight	36. four	36. five	36. four
37. five	37. ten	37. five	37. ten	37. eight	37. five	37. five
38. nine	38. eight	38. three	38. nine	38. nine	38. nine	38. ten
39. one	39. five	39. eight	39. three	39. six	39. three	39. nine
40. ten	40. two	40. one	40. nine	40. eight	40. seven	40. nine

DAY 8	DAY 9	DAY 10	DAY 11	DAY 12	DAY 13	DAY 14
1. two	1. eight	1. eight	1. five	1. four	1. seven	1. seven
2. five	2. three	2. five	2. seven	2. five	2. five	2. seven
3. five	3. eight	3. eight	3. seven	3. eight	3. three	3. five
4. seven	4. seven	4. six	4. five	4. eight	4. seven	4. four
5. nine	5. seven	5. five	5. nine	5. six	5. eight	5. four
6. six	6. six	6. nine	6. eight	6. eight	6. nine	6. five
7. five	7. five	7. eight	7. eight	7. nine	7. nine	7. five
8. eight	8. ten	8. eight	8. five	8. three	8. five	8. five
9. three	9. five	9. five	9. seven	9. six	9. ten	9. eight
10. ten	10. seven	10. five	10. two	10. four	10. seven	10. eight
11. four	11. six	11. three	11. nine	11. seven	11. ten	11. eight
12. four	12. five	12. two	12. eight	12. seven	12. six	12. six
13. three	13. three	13. ten	13. nine	13. ten	13. nine	13. four
14. five	14. ten	14. five	14. seven	14. six	14. seven	14. seven
15. four	15. eight	15. four	15. seven	15. eight	15. six	15. four
16. six	16. four	16. nine	16. seven	16. four	16. one	16. nine
17. nine	17. eight	17. eight	17. seven	17. two	17. seven	17. four
18. five	18. ten	18. ten	18. six	18. three	18. five	18. three
19. six	19. seven	19. seven	19. six	19. three	19. ten	19. three
20. six	20. six	20. five	20. two	20. three	20. nine	20. seven
21. six	21. eight	21. nine	21. six	21. five	21. seven	21. seven
22. six	22. nine	22. ten	22. four	22. four	22. four	22. two
23. seven	23. nine	23. ten	23. four	23. ten	23. ten	23. three
24. ten	24. four	24. four	24. five	24. seven	24. six	24. ten
25. four	25. three	25. five	25. three	25. three	25. seven	25. eight
26. three	26. ten	26. four	26. seven	26. ten	26. eight	26. ten
27. four	27. six	27. five	27. ten	27. three	27. nine	27. ten
28. three	28. three	28. two	28. four	28. six	28. five	28. one
29. ten	29. ten	29. ten	29. five	29. one	29. seven	29. four
30. eight	30. six	30. three	30. seven	30. five	30. nine	30. eight
31. nine	31. four	31. ten	31. six	31. three	31. four	31. ten
32. six	32. nine	32. seven	32. seven	32. five	32. ten	32. five
33. one	33. four	33. nine	33. ten	33. six	33. four	33. three
34. three	34. eight	34. six	34. two	34. six	34. three	34. four
35. eight	35. nine	35. three	35. seven	35. nine	35. three	35. one
36. ten	36. five	36. four	36. four	36. three	36. ten	36. eight
37. five	37. nine	37. seven	37. six	37. nine	37. five	37. seven
38. nine	38. seven	38. two	38. five	38. five	38. three	38. ten
39. nine	39. nine	39. eight	39. eight	39. nine	39. six	39. nine
40. two	40. five	40. seven	40. nine	40. eight	40. nine	40. three

DAY 15	DAY 16	DAY 17	DAY 18	DAY 19	DAY 20	DAY 21
1. ten	1. nine	1. five	1. eight	1. seven	1. four	1. three
2. nine	2. seven	2. six	2. zero	2. eight	2. five	2. one
3. ten	3. ten	3. two	3. one	3. four	3. ten	3. nine
4. four	4. nine	4. nine	4. six	4. nine	4. ten	4. nine
5. six	5. nine	5. seven	5. ten	5. nine	5. six	5. eight
6. six	6. nine	6. five	6. seven	6. eight	6. four	6. four
7. four	7. two	7. three	7. five	7. two	7. eight	7. eight
8. six	8. six	8. five	8. three	8. seven	8. nine	8. seven
9. seven	9. one	9. nine	9. five	9. eight	9. four	9. seven
10. ten	10. one	10. six	10. four	10. four	10. ten	10. six
11. nine	11. eight	11. three	11. ten	11. five	11. eight	11. five
12. four	12. five	12. one	12. six	12. ten	12. five	12. eight
13. ten	13. ten	13. four	13. eight	13. eight	13. nine	13. four
14. ten	14. one	14. four	14. nine	14. nine	14. eight	14. eight
15. seven	15. eight	15. nine	15. eight	15. two	15. ten	15. ten
16. three	16. three	16. five	16. seven	16. eight	16. five	16. three
17. ten	17. six	17. three	17. four	17. three	17. six	17. two
18. four	18. eight	18. two	18. six	18. four	18. three	18. nine
19. five	19. three	19. eight	19. two	19. five	19. three	19. five
20. eight	20. four	20. seven	20. nine	20. eight	20. two	20. four
21. four	21. one	21. three	21. four	21. eight	21. nine	21. two
22. nine	22. seven	22. eight	22. five	22. four	22. ten	22. eight
23. two	23. three	23. seven	23. eight	23. five	23. three	23. two
24. six	24. three	24. two	24. three	24. eight	24. nine	24. six
25. six	25. three	25. ten	25. nine	25. nine	25. three	25. five
26. ten	26. six	26. four	26. eight	26. ten	26. one	26. seven
27. nine	27. four	27. nine	27. five	27. four	27. three	27. five
28. four	28. seven	28. four	28. three	28. five	28. seven	28. three
29. nine	29. nine	29. six	29. six	29. ten	29. eight	29. six
30. one	30. nine	30. five	30. five	30. nine	30. eight	30. seven
31. four	31. ten	31. one	31. six	31. five	31. eight	31. four
32. five	32. nine	32. five	32. seven	32. four	32. six	32. two
33. five	33. five	33. six	33. two	33. six	33. three	33. five
34. seven	34. one	34. one	34. three	34. three	34. six	34. two
35. two	35. eight	35. two	35. seven	35. one	35. nine	35. seven
36. five	36. ten	36. seven	36. one	36. three	36. nine	36. six
37. eight	37. eight	37. five	37. seven	37. seven	37. four	37. four
38. ten	38. nine	38. eight	38. two	38. seven	38. four	38. nine
39. ten	39. six	39. eight	39. eight	39. two	39. two	39. eight
40. four	40. nine	40. seven	40. eight	40. nine	40. six	40. five

DAY 22	DAY 23	DAY 24	DAY 25	DAY 26	DAY 27	DAY 28
1. eight	1. ten	1. eight	1. four	1. four	1. nine	1. seven
2. seven	2. six	2. five	2. seven	2. nine	2. one	2. four
3. three	3. two	3. three	3. one	3. one	3. nine	3. seven
4. four	4. eight	4. eight	4. four	4. one	4. five	4. two
5. eight	5. three	5. two	5. nine	5. five	5. eight	5. eight
6. four	6. ten	6. nine	6. nine	6. three	6. one	6. ten
7. four	7. two	7. eight	7. four	7. nine	7. six	7. eight
8. two	8. nine	8. six	8. nine	8. three	8. five	8. nine
9. nine	9. eight	9. nine	9. two	9. four	9. two	9. six
10. two	10. eight	10. nine	10. four	10. seven	10. six	10. four
11. ten	11. three	11. three	11. two	11. six	11. three	11. seven
12. one	12. two	12. seven	12. nine	12. three	12. seven	12. ten
13. nine	13. three	13. eight	13. five	13. nine	13. nine	13. one
14. two	14. three	14. four	14. three	14. one	14. eight	14. six
15. eight	15. three	15. four	15. ten	15. eight	15. three	15. two
16. three	16. seven	16. six	16. four	16. four	16. nine	16. four
17. eight	17. six	17. four	17. four	17. eight	17. three	17. two
18. three	18. ten	18. one	18. four	18. three	18. seven	18. four
19. two	19. four	19. five	19. eight	19. six	19. six	19. eight
20. four	20. one	20. six	20. one	20. five	20. two	20. two
21. five	21. eight	21. three	21. eight	21. seven	21. five	21. eight
22. four	22. six	22. five	22. five	22. three	22. eight	22. six
23. zero	23. seven	23. four	23. six	23. nine	23. eight	23. six
24. six	24. three	24. one	24. two	24. nine	24. ten	24. four
25. seven	25. nine	25. six	25. seven	25. four	25. six	25. three
26. eight	26. two	26. three	26. seven	26. two	26. one	26. five
27. nine	27. three	27. one	27. four	27. eight	27. nine	27. five
28. five	28. two	28. seven	28. nine	28. one	28. one	28. eight
29. ten	29. one	29. five	29. eight	29. four	29. six	29. six
30. eight	30. two	30. four	30. seven	30. nine	30. five	30. four
31. four	31. seven	31. six	31. ten	31. five	31. three	31. seven
32. one	32. five	32. nine	32. six	32. one	32. five	32. six
33. three	33. three	33. eight	33. six	33. six	33. three	33. ten
34. two	34. eight	34. five	34. five	34. eight	34. nine	34. four
35. ten	35. five	35. seven	35. five	35. five	35. eight	35. two
36. three	36. five	36. seven	36. five	36. seven	36. four	36. two
37. six	37. four	37. two	37. seven	37. six	37. six	37. nine
38. three	38. nine	38. eight	38. eight	38. three	38. six	38. five
39. nine	39. nine	39. six	39. three	39. six	39. four	39. ten
40. eight	40. six	40. eight	40. three	40. five	40. one	40. three

THE BRAIN FUNCTION TESTS

PART I

Memory Function Test

For each memory test, take 2 minutes to memorize the corresponding list of words. Wait 30 seconds and then write down as many as you recall in 120 seconds. Your score is the number of correct responses. The maximum score is 25. Record your score on the Memory Function Test Record on page 174. The score for week 0 represents your baseline memory status. Repeat this test every 4 weeks in the same fashion, recording your score on the graph. That way you will be able to compare results with your baseline performance and graph your progress.

Week 0 (baseline)

SHADOW	PICTURE	APPLE	CHAIR	LOUNGE
PLATE	DRAMA	SHOVEL	LEVEL	HAMMER
OCEAN	SUNSET	TROMBONE	SOFA	BUREAU
HAZARD	ASPHALT	MOTOR	STAPLE	PLANE
PORTAL	VINTAGE	STORM	PORTICO	BIFOCAL

Week 4

FOREST	TABLE	BUREAU	ASPHALT	SIGNAL
WINTER	MELON	QUARTER	BEACH	TARGET
BALCONY	AIRPLANE	TELEPHONE	STRENGTH	PROBLEM
CAMERA	STAMP	PRODUCT	SEASHORE	PAPER
MARKET	COUNTRY	CAMPER	CHILDREN	HAMMER

Week 8

GUITAR	COFFEE	TREADMILL	SAUCER	PORCH
CHAPTER	FORMAT	DIVER	MIDGET	HANGER
TODAY	WINDOW	PROBLEM	ENGINE	ROBOT
STUBBORN	FOREHEAD	SCHOOL	SIEVE	BUCKLE
RIVER	CLOSET	BUSINESS	CAMERA	BASKET

Week 12

SHOULDER	VILLAGE	ADULT	FASHION	HOMEWORK
CIRCULAR	TROUBLE	AMBER	COUNTER	BATTERY
PLATEAU	ANVIL	BASKET	COLUMN	AISLE
PENCIL	TRACTOR	DINNER	CHAMBER	CIRCLE
TRAVEL	PARSLEY	LETTER	SUNSET	SYSTEM

Week 16

MISSION	PRIVATE	COURT	STRONG	DELETE
SERIES	COLOR	CORNER	BASEMENT	TASSEL
FRAME	SKYLINE	CLIFF	LAMP	CLOTH
SPREAD	NUMBER	PROBLEM	TICKET	RAPID
SCARF	PIZZA	SPEAKER	CLIFF	TULIP

Week 20

CLOSET	SHOWER	RECORD	SIMPLE	BOUQUET
CRANE	VISTA	LUMBER	MARKET	BORDER
PULLEY	TRAFFIC	CHORUS	BASEMENT	SCISSORS
UMBRELLA	HARDWARE	SLOGAN	TRADE	PARDON
GARDEN	ELECTRIC	TANDEM	BRIGADE	MATERIAL

Week 24

SIDEWALK	SKYLIGHT	ELASTIC	BUSINESS	ORCHESTRA
AXLE	PANTRY	CABINET	CANYON	BORDER
BOULDER	LAUNDRY	ISLAND	PROBLEM	JEWEL
COLUMN	ORDER	TRAM	DELETE	SURVEY
CARPOOL	SCHEDULE	PICTURE	AROMA	DESSERT

Week 28

FRAME	ARTIST	BUSINESS	DESIGN	AIRPORT
STREAM	SALAD	PARDON	CIRCLE	COPY
CURB	DRIVE	ROBBERY	CONTRACT	SURVIVE
VIDEO	PALACE	CAMPFIRE	STORY	TISSUE
SHELTER	HELMET	NECKLACE	BUCKET	SEWER

Week 32

CARPET	PADDLE	MEMORY	ROLLER	HANDLE
ORDER	FLOOR	PARCEL	TIRED	CHEESE
CREATE	IMPRESS	TRAUMA	STATION	WATER
ZEBRA	FIELD	CANDY	PATIO	SURROUND
SHORE	BOUNDARY	MORNING	THEORY	SILENCE

Week 36

BOTTLE	GRANT	EXTREME	GUTTER	MISSILE
HELMET	TREND	MARBLE	RECORD	CLOSET
FORMAL	QUALITY	CHANNEL	ANIMAL	PILLOW
CANDLE	DONUT	STAMP	GARAGE	CONTROL
DRAMA	STATION	FRAME	IMPULSE	INVEST

Week 40

CRADLE	HOUSE	JACKET	NORMAL	HEDGE
FOREST	ARRIVE	HOTEL	BRANCH	CANOE
FRAME	HANGAR	BRIDGE	ROCKET	STRIKE
COVER	TOPPLE	NEUTRAL	COARSE	DOUBT
NECKLACE	GUARD	LITTLE	PASTA	TORCH

Week 44

RANGER	SPARE	BULLET	PREDICT	SCANDAL
TENT	CATTLE	STORM	AVERAGE	CORPORATE
TARNISH	COMMUTE	MEETING	CONNECT	SALAD
STORAGE	UNDER	VELVET	EXTERNAL	CORRECT
ARRANGE	CONTROL	ASIDE	BALANCE	PENCIL

Week 48

COMPASS	STUDY	SMART	BOTTLE	REMIND
SPRINT	CURRENT	CHEESE	ABOUT	COLLECT
STRAND	CHURCH	BENEATH	COACH	PLANK
SPRING	VANDAL	EMPIRE	FINGER	CEREAL
DRINK	CASTLE	SALAMI	CURVE	PRAYER

Week 52

SINGLE	QUART	GRAND	JOKER	DIRTY
SAND	SURVIVE	CRIMP	DANGER	ABOUT
UNDER	TRANSIT	STYLE	GRASS	BREATHE
CRUNCH	SHIFT	TRUNK	ANKLE	ESTATE
GOOSE	TUNNEL	PROVIDE	STRANGE	SILENCE

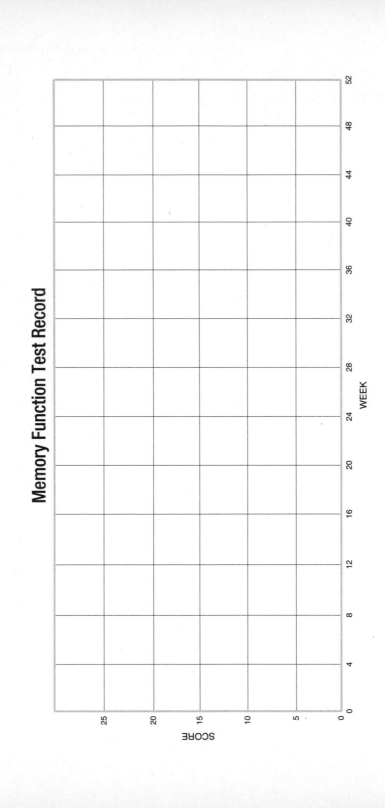

Memory Function Test Record

THE MEMORY FUNCTION TEST RECORD

Each month (baseline, week 4, week 8, and so on) record the number of words you correctly recalled by placing a point on the graph that corresponds to the test result. Join the dots to create a graph of your progress.

PART II

The Trail-Making Test

The Trail-Making Test is a variant of a test by the same name that was developed by the U.S. Army. It is designed to see how flexible your thinking is by forcing you to jump back and forth from numbers to letters while simultaneously keeping track of where you are in each sequence. To perform the test, take a pencil and connect the items sequentially without raising your pencil off the paper. You are to alternate from numbers to letters as follows: 1-A-2-B-3-C-4-D and so on to 10 and J, until you have completed the test. Your score is the time it takes to complete the test. You will need a stopwatch or a clock with a second hand to determine your score. After completing each test, record your score in the Trail-Making Test Record. To get you started, the number 1 has been printed in bold type and underlined (**1**) for easy identification.

You are to complete the week 0 version of the Trail-Making Test before starting the Mental Gymnastics portion of the Brain Trust Program to establish a baseline level of performance. Every 4 weeks you will complete a different version of the Trail-Making Test (week 4, week 8, and so on).

Week 0 (Baseline)   Time_____

J

2

B

8

A   10   J

4

H

6

F   7

9   I

C   D

<u>1</u>

E

G

3

5

Week 4   Time_____

6

1

J

8

I   H

5

3

A

E

F

G

2

C

D   B

7   9

4

10

Week 8   Time_____

E

10

B   9

H

8

6

A   2   J

3

D

4

5

F   G   I

C

<u>1</u>

7

Week 12   Time_____

2

E

4

8

C

A

B

6

1

H

10

F

G

5

3

7

J

I

D

9

Week 16   Time_____

6   J

1   C

8

4

7

I

10

E

F

3   A   D

9

5

G

2

B   H

Week 20 Time_____

2   3
                    9
        G
                        7

4
            J

                1
        B
    H

6
        I   C   F
    D
                            5
    E   8
                    10
            A

Week 24   Time_____

G   4

B

2

6

9

C

F

3   5

8

D

A

7

10   H

I

1

E

J

Week 28   Time_____

G   5

        9

2

            A   J

                                    F

    7   E

                    4   8

    B

                            C

                        10

1

            6   I

    H

                D

                                3

Week 32   Time_____

7

8

D

B

F

G

3

H

4

9

A

E

2

6

J

C

5

<u>1</u>

10

I

Week 36 Time_____

7

A   D

4   H

J

G

C

5

1

I

E

8   B   F

9

2   3

10

6

Week 40   Time_____

I

5

J

7

4

10

E

9

1

B

6

C

D

H

G

A

3

2

F

8

Week 44   Time_____

4

F

3

G

9

10

D

1

C

7

A

H

6

B

I

5

8

2

E

J

Week 48   Time_____

C

1

I

4

A   J

6
H

G
B

D

E

9

3

8

F
10

5

2

7

H

8

B

D   C

6

3

F

A   G

9

10

5

4

2   J

1

I   E

7

THE TRAIL-MAKING TEST RECORD

Plot your time on the Trail-Making Test Record every 4 weeks (week 0, week 4, week 8, and so on) and connect the dots to graph your progress.

Trail-Making Test Record

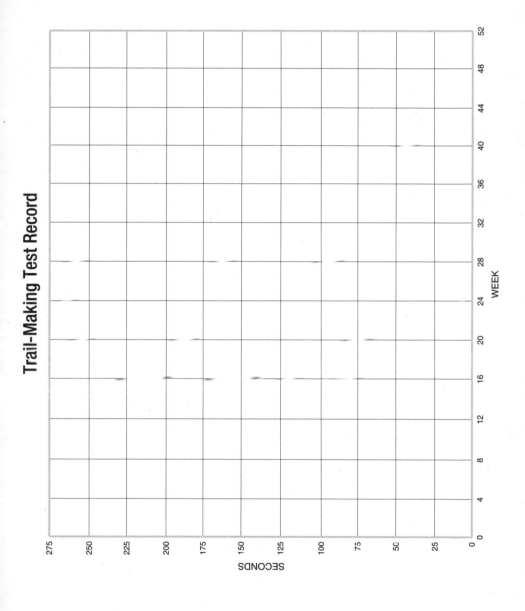

Novel Applications of the Brain Trust Program

Good Brains Gone Bad: Menopause, Migraine, Dimming of the Senses, and Alzheimer's Disease

Science tells us that the brain you start with dictates to a large extent the brain you'll be left with in old age. An obvious statement to be sure; clearly some people are born with greater brain wattage than others and some have more left at the end. But it's more than just the luck of the genetic draw that determines brain function, although that is clearly one component. It also, and perhaps mainly, has to do with how well you nourish what you start with. By that, I mean not only nourishment with the nutrient raw materials from food but also the nourishment of learning and mental stimulation of all types that promotes the formation of rich interconnections within the brain. Research supports the notion that those with greater brain volume and higher levels of education are much less likely to suffer substantial memory decline, including even Alzheimer's disease, with age.

Yet, regardless of how robust and well connected a brain we have in our youth or prime, age will take its toll to a greater or lesser degree, depending on how vigorously we work to preserve its function throughout life—that's what the Brain Trust Program is all about. But even the healthiest and most agile brain may be subject to disabilities of clear thinking—brain fog, if you will—depression, anxiety, or other types of malfunction. Let's take a look at two of the most common ones: menopause and migraines.

Hormones, Hot Flashes, and Brain Fog

Doctors call them symptoms of vasomotor instability, those unpleasant sensations of warmth, sweating, and redness that flush abruptly from chest to neck to head when blood vessels in the skin suddenly dilate. Most people know them as hot flashes or night sweats; if you've ever had one, you probably call them something worse. Even when you're just in the same room with someone who suffers from them, you can readily appreciate the tremendous discomfort endured by—in some estimates—75 percent of women as they enter their menopausal years.

Research has linked an abrupt drop in reproductive hormone levels, whether as a consequence of natural menopause or the result of surgery, with vasomotor instability. Survivors of breast and ovarian cancer are especially vulnerable to hot flash symptoms. While you're probably familiar with surgical menopause caused by removal of the ovaries in women, it might surprise you to know that men can suffer from hot flashes as well! Removal of the testes or treatment with testosterone-blocking drugs, such as those used to treat prostate cancer, can trigger hot flashes in men that produce the same symptoms women suffer from.

It is interesting that there isn't a significant correlation between how much estrogen is in the blood and the development of hot flash symptoms, meaning that estrogen levels alone can't explain them; something else is clearly at work. After all, young girls who have not yet reached puberty have low levels of estrogen but don't have hot flashes. So what gives? It appears that for symptoms to develop, the body must first have become used to having estrogen around for a prolonged stretch of time. The subsequent withdrawal of estrogen, once the body has become used to it, can then trigger the development of hot flashes in a manner not entirely unlike withdrawal from narcotic addition.

In an attempt to understand this process, Dr. James Simpkins and his colleagues at the University of Florida College of Pharmacy developed an animal model, based on morphine-addicted rats, designed to mimic the symptoms associated with hot flashes. Once the rats had become accustomed to a certain level of morphine, Simpkins injected them with a morphine-blocking drug to throw them quickly into morphine withdrawal; then he monitored them carefully to see what would happen. What he observed was the rat equivalent of a hot flash: a strong increase in the temperature of their tail skin, a rapid rise in their heart rate, and the elevation of the same hormone (luteinizing hormone, or LH) that rises in women when estrogen levels fall. And even more amazing, giving estrogen to these morphine-addicted rats stopped their withdrawal symptoms, just as giving estrogen to women alleviates theirs.

Simpkins's experiments suggest that chronic estrogen exposure and chronic narcotic exposure, as different as they clearly are, may influence the brain in similar ways; in both situations, the brain gets used to the regular presence of a substance and responds to its abrupt removal in much the same fashion. In this light, the symptoms of menopause could be viewed as the brain's response to life without estrogen. Scientists have recently pinpointed a region of the brain as a potential culprit in the development of menopausal symptoms. When hot flashes occur, so does excessive electrical firing of brain cells in the hypothalamus, a part of the brain intimately involved in regulation of appetite, temperature, and response to stress. A growing body of evidence supports the notion that hot flashes occur because the hypothalamus becomes extraordinarily sensitive to tiny increases in body temperature. But what causes the temperature increase to begin with?

To answer that question, I turn again to Simpkins and his rats. He performed an experiment designed to test what happened when the rats' brains were blocked from getting enough glucose, or blood sugar. This was achieved by giving the animals a substance called 2-deoxy-D-glucose (2DG), which is almost identical to glucose, the brain's main energy source, with one critical difference: 2DG can't be turned into energy. Giving a slug of 2DG to a rat's brain causes an instant energy crisis throughout the brain, including the hypothalamus, and reliably produces symptoms identical to a hot flash. This observation suggests a link between the production of hot flashes and a glucose shortage in the hypothalamus. Another interesting note that further supports the association among low estrogen, glucose shortage, and narcotic withdrawal is that when Simpkins gave glucose along with the morphine-blocking drug to the rats, the animals' symptoms of withdrawal were reduced. Upon further investigation, Simpkins found that the hot flashes in rats given 2DG occurred in concert with a rise in a particular brain-signaling chemical called norepinephrine (NE) in the hypothalamus. His findings support the contention that an energy shortfall in the brain cells, due to inadequate glucose, triggers hot flashes—at least in rats.

Evidence from human research supports this connection, too. A study of women just entering their menopausal years reported that the timing of hot flashes frequently coincided with periods of low blood sugar seen a few hours after eating. Another study found a similar association between falling glucose and hot flashes; experimentally raising the blood sugar level significantly reduced the symptoms. What does all this have to do with brain heath and improving memory? Plenty!

During hot flash episodes, women—unlike rats—can tell us how they feel, and they frequently describe various brain or nervous system symptoms such as anxiety, difficulty with focus or attention, problems learning new information, forgetfulness, insomnia, depression, and mood swings. Medical research suggests that the brain fog, mood swings, and other symptoms women sometimes experience during their reproductive decline relate more to the hormonal transition rather than simply to aging.

The explanation is quite clear. Blood sugar gets ferried into the brain on a little shuttle called a transporter. This mechanism is the main way blood sugar reaches the brain cells. Estrogen tells the brain cells to make more of these sugar shuttles. In fact, under the influence of estrogen, the shuttle system ferries a whopping 40 percent more blood sugar across the blood–brain barrier and into brain cells than in the absence of estrogen. When estrogen levels decline, shuttling of glucose into the brain decreases, the brain cells become relatively starved for energy, and the brain cells in the hypothalamus must do something to fix the fuel shortage. The hypothalamus, for its part, complies by stepping up the release of norepinephrine, which acts to raise the level of sugar in the blood, to raise the heart rate, and to raise the body temperature. The hot flash, then, is a specific outward sign of the brain's trying to protect itself from blood sugar starvation!

Shortage of glucose bedevils the brain cells in two ways. First, it creates an energy deficit or brown out, with the consequences described earlier. Researchers once thought that the failure to generate enough energy directly damaged the brain cells. Now, however, evidence points to a second cause: The energy deficit produces a buildup of a brain-signaling chemical called glutamate. Glutamate acts to stimulate the brain cells, which in the right amount at the right time is critical to their normal function. However, when excess glutamate spurs the brain cells to work harder, they naturally require more energy. When the brain cell is already energy deprived, the buildup of glutamate places an added demand on the burdened system. Just as with the electricity to your home, a spike of use that exceeds supply can blow out the circuits. In the case of the brain cell, the combination of rising energy demand and falling supply can lead to damage or even cell death. If the process continues year after year, the loss of brain cells will lead to brain fog and even worse degrees of memory loss.

The good news is that research has shown that replacing reproductive hormones during this menopausal transition pays significant rewards later in life. Women who received hormone-replacement therapy during early menopause had a 64 percent decrease in their risk for developing significant memory impairment later in life. This research supports the position that taking hormone replacement for the short term—for just a few years only at the beginning of the menopausal transition—can both alleviate uncomfortable physical symptoms in many women and protect the brain as well.

Unfortunately, there appears to be no protective benefit to the brain if replacement isn't begun until after menopause is complete. The question of whether or not to take hormones (even short term) rests with the individual and her physician. Hormone replacement simply isn't for everybody; unfortunately, it's particularly not for breast and ovarian cancer survivors, who are often the very group most affected by hot flashes. What else, then, can sufferers do to curtail hot flashes and lift the brain fog that accompanies them?

THE METABOLIC APPROACH TO HOT FLASH THERAPY

As we learned, emerging data suggest that as estrogen levels decline, so does the brain's ability to shuttle glucose across the blood–brain barrier and into its cells for energy. Somehow, the hot flash may function as a countermeasure on the part of the energy-starved brain to try to alleviate the situation by raising the blood sugar level. If indeed this is the case, it would seem logical that a solution to the problem might be to either make the shuttle work better to help the blood sugar cross into the brain more easily or to find an alternative fuel for the brain to free it from its dependence on glucose. How can this be done? The dietary treatment for an uncommon form of childhood epilepsy offers insight. A rare genetic disorder that causes developmental delays and epilepsy in children also involves the shuttle mechanism that ferries glucose across the blood–brain barrier. These children's brains make faulty shuttles, which fail to properly move glucose into their brains. As a consequence, the blood sugar level in their brain tissue is very low, causing their symptoms. A special diet—the same one employed by neurologists for decades to control severe seizure disorders of other types in children—has emerged as the treatment of choice for this genetic deficiency of sugar shuttles. The ketogenic diet, as it's called, provides the brain with ketone bodies (which don't happen to require the use of the faulty shuttles) as an alternative fuel source to blood sugar. The diet works when nothing else, including potent medications, will because the brain cells don't need glucose per se but the energy it represents.

Ketone bodies, or simply ketones, are the natural by-products of fat burning; they're basically partially burned fats. We all produce them every night while we sleep, if we go without eating for a prolonged period, or when we restrict dietary carbohydrates. Many tissues, including the heart, prefer them to glucose as the fuel of choice. Ketones are particularly useful for children with the faulty sugar shuttle disorder because they cross the blood–brain barrier via a different shuttle system. Once in the brain, the ketones stoke the cellular furnaces, providing fuel for the energy-starved brain cells.

The same situation we find in children with this form of epilepsy occurs in the brains of women at the beginning of menopause, although clearly to a much lesser degree. For the women, inadequate estrogen leads to fewer sugar shuttles, which leads to less glucose being available to the brain cells, which leads to an energy crisis, which leads to a surge of NE, which leads to a hot flash in an effort to raise the low sugar level. You could call what's happening in both these cases—and in point of fact in other thought process and memory disorders, such as Alzheimer's disease—brain starvation. Simply put, the brain can't manage its energy budget; it can't create enough energy to meet its needs. This deficit produces rolling brown outs in the brain, leading to seizures in children with the rare genetic disorder and to brain fog and hot flashes in perimenopausal women.

Because the cause of these symptoms is similar, so is the treatment. A few simple dietary changes can provide the alternative fuel source, prevent the energy crisis in the brain cells, and interrupt the whole cascade that culminates in the hot flash. It can be accomplished without side effects, without resorting to medications, and without replacing hormones!

To provide a ready supply of alternative fuel to the brain, I recommend that women on the cusp of menopause who have begun to suffer hot flashes, foggy thinking, or mood swings carefully follow the basic Brain Trust Program (outlined in Chapters 4, 5, and 6) and take further care to avoid any excess starch or sugar. Women who rely primarily on meat, fish, poultry, eggs, cheese, nuts, fresh low-sugar fruits, greens, and low-starch vegetables and limit their intake of breads, cereals, pasta, potatoes, sodas, and sweets will be better able to produce the ketones that serve as an alternate brain fuel. In addition, these women should supplement their diets with a specific mixture of healthy oils that their bodies can quickly and effectively turn into ketones. This Ketogenic Cocktail (see page 203) functions like rocket fuel for the brain.

The main components of the cocktail are as follows:

- **MEDIUM-CHAIN TRIGLYCERIDE (MCT) OIL.** You probably think of triglycerides as being one of the fats in your blood, which they indeed are. Triglycerides are the storage form of fat, a very high octane fuel source, made of long chains of carbon atoms hooked together in various lengths. The number of carbon links in the chain determines whether the molecules are called short-chain, long-chain, or medium-chain triglycerides. The body can readily turn the medium-length chains into ketones for energy, a notion body builders and athletes caught onto long ago. That is why you'll find MCT oil in health food stores and in the health and nutritional supplement aisle of your grocery store or pharmacy. MCT oil is quite stable, so much so that even after having been opened, it does not need to be refrigerated or kept away from light.

- **FLAXSEED OIL.** The chief component of flaxseed oil is the long-chain omega-3 fatty acid called α-linolenic acid (ALA). The body can take this oil and turn a tiny bit of it (about 1 percent) into decosahexanoic acid (DHA), one of the essential fatty acids found in fish oil (discussed in Chapter 5). The vast bulk of ALA, however, gets burned for energy, and this process helps promote ketone formation. You'll find flaxseed oil in the refrigerated case of your local health food store, natural grocer, or pharmacy. To keep it from going rancid, flaxseed oil must be protected from prolonged exposure to light, heat, and air; keep it tightly capped in the refrigerator. Buy the smallest available size bottle and use it quickly.

- **EICOSAPENTANOIC ACID (EPA).** Recent research indicates that EPA, an essential fat found naturally along with DHA in cold-water fish and krill, can speed up the burning of long-chain triglycerides for energy and thereby improve the generation of ketones to fuel the brain. Like flaxseed oil, EPA is delicate and highly prone to rancidity. Keep bottles or capsules of fish oil, or EPA/DHA extracted from fish oil, refrigerated and protected from light, heat, and air. When fresh, the product doesn't taste fishy; if it does, throw it out and replace it with a new bottle. Krill oil, because of its phosphatide chemical linkage (discussed in Chapter 5) does not require refrigeration; it should be kept cool, dry, and protected from direct light but not refrigerated.

BOX 7.1. Ketogenic Cocktail

Take whole cocktail one to three times per day.

1–2 tablespoons MCT oil (about 15 grams/tablespoon)
1 teaspoon to 1 tablespoon flaxseed oil
50 mg EPA

As you now know, the brief episodes of energy brown out experienced along with hot flashes allow an excess of the brain chemical glutamate to accumulate. This brain chemical excites the cells, putting an added energy demand on an already strained system. If left unchecked, the excitatory overload can damage or even destroy the brain cells. As an added measure of protection against cellular overstimulation, I suggest that women experiencing menopausal symptoms should also increase the daily amounts of several specific supplements, some of which I recommended at slightly lower doses in Chapter 5.

The first is magnesium, which isn't well absorbed and in high doses can sometimes cause mild diarrhea. If intestinal tolerance will permit it, increase your intake of magnesium to a daily total of 800 milligrams taken in two equal-400 milligram doses. Increase the dose of huperzine A to 75 micrograms twice a day. Include vinpocetine at a daily dose of 5 milligrams twice a day. This group of supplements helps curb excitation in the brain. Several other supplements have proven helpful to increase brain relaxation. These include γ-aminobutyric acid (GABA) (a glutamate antagonist), taurine, and

> BOX 7.2. **Anti-Excitatory Cocktail**
>
> **Take whole cocktail twice per day.**
>
> 400 milligrams magnesium   10 milligrams thiamin
>
> 75 micrograms huperzine A   50 milligrams GABA
>
> 5 milligrams vinpocetine   1 gram taurine
>
> **Plus 1 milligram melatonin at bedtime**

melatonin. I recommend taking 50 milligrams of GABA twice a day, 1 gram of taurine twice a day, and 1 milligram of melatonin just before bedtime. In addition to thiamin, these supplements work in concert to relax and calm the brain and form the core of what I call the Anti-Excitatory Cocktail (see above).

By following the correct diet and taking the Ketogenic Cocktail and the Anti-Excitatory Cocktail, you will feel better, think straighter, and stop hot flashes in their tracks.

Migraine Headaches

It may surprise you to learn that the brain feels no pain. Like all neurosurgeons, I have done extensive brain surgeries on many patients while they were awake, comfortable, and talking to me. Strange as it sounds, it's a technique that brain surgeons must sometimes use when operating on tumors or blood vessel irregularities in and around the speech centers of the brain. But, if the brain can't feel pain, then why do we experience headaches? Clearly, something in the head, other than the brain itself, hurts. And in fact, there are a number of pain-sensitive tissues in the head responsible for the suffering we call a headache.

Headaches come in many types, some of them painful but not serious; others, such as the migraine headache, totally disabling, at least temporarily. An estimated 10 to 15 percent of people worldwide suffer from migraines, the (usually) one-sided, throbbing headache often accompanied by nausea; vomiting; and sensitivity to light, noise, and motion. The interesting thing about migraines is that although the brain can't feel pain, it turns out to be the actual cause of this type of headache, a notion we'll explore momentarily. But first, let's back up for a little history.

Migraines are nothing new; they've been recognized and treated by medical practitioners for thousands of years. The earliest known medical reference to them—the Ebers papyrus, dating to about 1550 B.C.E., from Thebes, Egypt—mentions several remedies for "suffering in half the head" (the classic migraine pattern we know today), including one that involved anointing the head with "the ashes from the burnt skull of a catfish." About 1,000 years later, the Greek physician Hippocrates first described the classic visual auras—the flashing lights, shiny shapes, spots, sparkles, colors, or halos drifting across the field of vision that warn about one in five sufferers that a migraine headache is on the horizon. Then, in the second century C.E., the Roman physician Galen coined the term *hemicrania* (meaning "half the head"), which later became the Old English word *megrim*, and then, finally, the French word *migraine* that we still use today. But what exactly is this type of headache?

A migraine originates entirely within the brain itself, painlessly, with a burst of unusual firing from one or more small clusters of brain cells. This signal then spreads in an expanding wave of electrical excitement across the surface of the brain, like the widening rings created by a pebble dropped into still water. If the initial burst occurs in the part of the brain that controls vision, the subsequent wave of electrical activity may be responsible for the auras (the flashing lights, shapes, and sparkles) in those people who experience them before developing the headache.

But what prompts the cluster of brain cells to become unusually excitable, hyperactive, and start firing in the first place? Research points to a buildup of calcium and sodium within the cells, and the cause of the buildup, once again, appears to be an energy-production deficit. As we've learned, to curb excessive excitation, the brain cells must be able to quickly push calcium and sodium back out of their interiors once the elements have done their jobs. However, that's an energy-intensive operation, and if the cell can't meet the demand, a focus of hyperexcitement blossoms.

The abnormal firing activity brought on by this relative power outage triggers the release of an array of compounds (some that cause inflammation, others that open or narrow arteries) into the fluid cushion that surrounds the brain and spinal cord. Once there, these compounds irritate the pain sensors of the trigeminal nerve, the main nerve that detects sensations such as pain in the tissues within the head that are able to feel pain (chiefly the blood vessels and the fibrous tissues that cover the brain). The current thinking is that irritation of the pain sensors on the surface of the blood vessels and brain coverings by these compounds causes migraine headache pain. Worse yet, instead of becoming accustomed to being bathed in the inflammatory compounds, with repeated migraine episodes the recurrent stimulation makes the nerve endings in these areas hyperirritable and all the more sensitive, such that the release of ever smaller amounts of inflammatory substances can bring on a headache. And for most migraine sufferers, an ever-growing list of foods or activities—chocolate, stress, alcohol, lack of sleep, hormonal fluctuations, and even certain cheeses—that seem to trigger an attack accompanies the increase in frequency. It can become a miserable and vicious circle of pain, and many migraine sufferers are helpless to break the cycle. But there is hope!

As noted, the most common reason brain cells become hyperexcitable is because they suffer an energy-production shortfall that leaves them without enough power to push calcium and sodium back out of their interiors. Although there are a number of prescription seizure medications that work to reduce brain cell excitability and are helpful in curtailing migraines, science now offers us another clue to a simpler remedy that should offer relief.

Sophisticated brain-scanning techniques have documented the presence of low magnesium levels in the brains of migraine patients. If this deficiency plays a role in triggering a migraine by permitting the buildup of excess calcium, then it would stand to reason that supplementation of magnesium to restore normal levels should help, because magnesium limits the flow of calcium into nerve cells. Research tells us that indeed this is so: Supplementing

BOX 7.3. Antimigraine Cocktail

Please note that the antimigraine cocktail represents the recommended total daily intake of these nutrients, to be taken in place of and *not in addition to* the amounts of these nutrients recommended in Chapter 5. Take this cocktail twice a day.

400 milligrams magnesium
1 gram taurine
100 milligrams coenzyme Q10
100 micrograms huperzine A
10 milligrams vinpocetine

Plus Ketogenic Cocktail (page 203) twice daily (if migraines are still problematic after a trial of the above cocktail)

with magnesium can help prevent migraines and can make them less painful and of shorter duration.

Similarly, supplementation with several other natural substances has shown promise. The amino acid taurine, for instance, has been shown to dampen the excitability of brain cells, a clear goal in migraine prevention. Vinpocetine, an herbal extract has been shown to block the sodium channel in much the same way that magnesium blocks calcium's entry. Huperzine A blocks the hyperexcitability caused by excess glutamate, another one of the excitatory brain chemicals. Together, these natural agents form an effective nutrient regimen (see Box 7.3 above) to reduce the frequency and severity of migraines.

In addition, to the general regimen of supplementation I recommend in Chapter 5 for optimal brain health, migraine sufferers may also need to increase their total daily doses of certain supplements to better guard against the energy shortfalls that can trigger migraines.

A DOCTOR'S LETTER

And finally, supplemental nutrients aside, the basic diet you eat can have a tremendous effect on the frequency and intensity of your migraines. Take a look at this most interesting case in point, the story of a long-term migraine sufferer, detailed by her husband, a physician, in a letter to the editor published in the medical journal *Headache*[1]:

My wife began having severe headaches in elementary school. The headaches worsened during her teenage years and were officially diagnosed as migraines. The family history is significant for severe migraines on the paternal side.

The migraines were described as a throbbing, burning, hot knife sensation in one temple. During her adulthood, the headaches progressed and were occurring many times a week. She tried multiple lifestyle changes without any change in the frequency of the headaches. Exercise, dieting, and two pregnancies did not alter the frequency. Numerous medications were prescribed by the neurologists over the years. . . . Imitrex 50 mg, Amerge 2.5 mg, and Fioricet.

In an effort to lose weight gained during pregnancy, [she] enrolled in a diet program under medical supervision . . . a modified fast, taking 3 to 4 high-protein, low-carbohydrate [200 calorie] shakes a day . . . [her] sole calorie source. Ketosis is induced . . . [and] a caloric restriction to 600 to 800 calories per day is maintained. . . .

After going into ketosis, my wife went from having almost daily headaches to being completely free of migraines. Her last migraine was in late April 2004. She maintained ketosis and the modified fast for almost 7 months and then went off her fast and began to eat regular foods. She has continued to be headache-free. She has now gone from daily migraines to going 14 months without an attack and has gradually

1. From R. S. Strahlman. "Can Ketosis Help Migraine Sufferers? A Case Report." *Headache* 46 (2006): 182.

reintroduced trigger foods such as alcohol and chocolate without getting a headache. [K]etosis appears to have cured my wife's migraines. . . . This letter is submitted with the hope of stimulating further research to confirm the benefits of a ketogenic diet on migraines."

An amazing story to be sure, but is it only that? Could there be a basis to believe that ketosis would curtail migraines just as it does hot flashes? Yes! Ketosis changes the way a brain cell handles substances, such as certain amino acids, that either excite it or calm it down, tipping the balance toward an overall calming effect on the brain. The benefit of the ketogenic diet to calm a hyperexcitable brain has been proven again and again over nearly a century as an effective treatment for young children with severe seizure disorders who fail to respond to medication.

It would make perfect sense that a ketogenic diet, such as the modified fast that benefited the doctor's wife, would reduce the frequency of migraine headaches. When you think about it, a seizure is one type of uncontrolled activity triggered by abnormal excitement that begins in a small group of brain cells and a migraine is generated by a slightly different type of uncontrolled burst of abnormal excitement in a similar group of brain cells.

If you are a migraine sufferer, you don't have to spend months on a very low calorie, modified fast under a doctor's care for a ketogenic diet to help you. Begin by following the complete Brain Trust Program guidelines for diet, supplements, and exercise; in many cases it may be all that's necessary. If you still suffer migraines even on the plan, I recommend that you follow the directions in Box 7.3.

Dimming of the Senses

The sensory organs—eyes, ears, nose, skin, and taste buds—may seem like a disparate group of unrelated body parts; but, in fact, they are all specialized extensions of the brain. The retina (a layer of cells in the back of the eye that allows us to see) is but a field of specialized endings of the optic nerve (the nerve that connects the eye to the brain). These nerve endings have the ability to convert the light waves that enter the eye into chemical messages and finally into electrical impulses that travel up the nerve to the occipital lobe (the part of the brain that allows us to see the signals that the eye receives) in the back of the brain.

The ear, at least the part visible from the outside, is nothing but a funnel to collect sound waves down to the eardrum, which converts those waves into mechanical energy to stimulate tiny hair-like nerve endings in the cochlea, the actual organ of hearing buried deep within the skull. The nerve endings in the cochlea are connected directly to nerve cells housed in the auditory processing regions of the temporal lobes of the brain. Same for the nose; it's a pair of funnels to draw air into the chambers in which lie the nerve endings of the olfactory nerve (the nerve of smell) which connects to various brain regions involved in the perception of odors.

Like the brain, with age, the sensory organs degenerate somewhat; and, as a consequence, our senses dim: We don't see as clearly, can't hear as well, and lose some of our ability to smell and taste. Like the brain, since the sensory organs are just specialized extensions of the brain cells, we can keep them healthy and preserve their function longer through feeding and caring for them properly.

For instance, one of the chief causes of blindness with aging (apart from diabetes, which is far and away number one) is macular degeneration, the death of nerve cells in the most critical part of the retina in the back of the eye. Let me hasten to distinguish this visual disorder of aging from the most common one that has nearly everyone over 40 reaching for the reading glasses: presbyopia, the inability to see up close objects clearly that comes to most of us. The need for reading glasses isn't brain related at all, but rather results from stiffening of the lens of the eye, which focuses the images we see onto the retina. To focus clearly up close the lens must be pliable so that the muscles that surround it can squeeze it to make it thicker or relax to make it thinner. When it's stiffened with age the mechanism simply doesn't work and, at least at this point, there isn't much we can do about it once presbyopia occurs.

As for the less common, but more serious macular degeneration, research has repeatedly shown that certain antioxidants and plant-derived compounds, particularly lutein and bilberry extract, can dramatically reduce the risk of developing macular degeneration and preserve vision longer. In addition to the nutritional and supplemental regimen prescribed as part of the Brain Trust Program, I also recommend that people with a family risk of macular degeneration supplement with these two compounds and protect their eyes from sun damage by wearing UV-blocking sunglasses or a broad-brimmed hat when they're out of doors in bright light. Another useful supplement on the market is called PreserVision, which contains vitamins C and E combined with zinc and copper.

The most frequent early complaint from people suffering from age-related hearing loss is an increasing difficulty in hearing conversations in a crowded room. The loss that occurs with age, called in medical parlance presbyacusis, involves the loss of higher frequency sounds, often in the range of the human voice, and is chiefly due to changes in the nerve cells, wrought in large part by exposure to loud noises over a lifetime. Throughout life in the urban world, except during sleep, nonstop noise assaults our ears: honking horns, squealing brakes, wailing sirens, concert crowds, and amplified music—which is now pumped via MP3 players directly into the ear canals of millions of people all day.

Excessive noise has been fingered as a culprit in overexciting the brain cells that make up the auditory (hearing) nerve. Excitation, as you'll recall from previous chapters, means that a large amount of the neurotransmitter glutamate bathes the cell, opening the door for the entry of a flood of calcium, which because it is toxic to the cells, must be pushed back out at enormous energy cost. The work of trying to push the calcium back out of the cells can overwhelm their energy-production capacity. When this occurs, calcium and its toxic message buildup within the vulnerable nerve cells. Under these conditions, brain cells can literally be excited to death by chronic excess noise. Over time, the net result is loss of the brain cells necessary for hearing. So what can be done besides donning OSHA-approved protective

BOX 7.4. **10-Item University of Pennsylvania Smell Identification Test**

The long version of UPSIT is widely used in research studies to assess abnormalities in odor identification. Deficits in odor identification and discrimination, especially when associated with unawareness of such loss of ability, are frequently linked with cognitive decline associated with development of neurofibrillary tangles, the pathological changes seen in patients with Alzheimer's disease. Remember that the sensory organs are quite literally direct extensions of the brain and, as such, often reflect its state of health and may be bellwethers for future changes. The major drawback of the full UPSIT test battery is that it requires a long and protracted examination. To maintain utility, but to enhance practicality, a subset of 10 items has been identified that retain the essence of the test while simultaneously and dramatically simplifying the administration of the odor profile. Those items are presented here.

For an olfactory test to be useful for early detection of certain types of mental decline, it must be sensitive to the earliest apparent changes, be short and easy to administer, and add significantly to current predictive risk factors. A family member may administer this test to a relative or friend in

hearing gear (or at least ear plugs) at the next Stones concert or turning down the volume on your iPod? As you learned in Chapter 5, you can protect the brain and nerve cells from within by slowing down the entry of calcium with extra magnesium, nature's own calcium channel blocker. Studies have documented that magnesium supplementation (400 mg per day) helps preserve hearing from the trauma wrought by overexcitation with noise.

Likewise, our ability to detect odors wanes as the years go by and is another example of good brains gone bad. Our sense of smell is seated in the most primitive parts of the brain. It was probably a great deal more important for survival in earlier eras of human existence than in modern times, when we relied on smell to warn us of the approach of predators or alerted us to the trail of game animals. Nowadays, although you might be tempted about 10 minutes once all the test items are collected. The results of the test in association with the loss of awareness of problems with the sense of smell are much better predictors of conversion to Alzheimer's disease or mental decline than low olfaction scores alone.

The 10 odors are menthol, clove, leather, strawberry, lilac, pineapple, smoke, soap, natural gas odor (rotten eggs), and lemon.

Since there is no kit, you must collect sources for these odors. Store them away from the subject. To conduct the test, blindfold the person and present each odor for 15 seconds. Wait 30 seconds after each response before presenting the next test odor.

Scores range from 0 to 10. A score of 10 means that all of the 10 test items were correctly identified. If 3 or more items are identified incorrectly, there is a fivefold increase in the risk of development of Alzheimer's Disease. Here it is important to note that any loss of olfaction related to local disease, such as sinusitis, has no predictive power. In addition, the results are meant to be interpreted in the broader perspective of a comprehensive medical evaluation.[2]

2. From M. H. Tabert, X. Liu, R. L. Doty, M. Serby, D. Zamora, A. H. Pelton, K. Marder, M. W. Alberts, Y. Stern, and D. P. Devanand. "A 10-Item Smell Identification Scale Related to Risk for Alzheimer's Disease." *Annals of Neurology* 58 (2005): 155–160.

to view the loss of sense of smell, which commonly affects older people, as a minor inconvenience, it can be dangerous in its own right as well as an early sign of potentially more serious trouble in store for the brain.

Say, for instance, that an older gentleman has lost his ability to smell the sulfurous odor of rotten eggs. You might be tempted, at first, to say "So what? Who wants to smell rotten eggs, anyway?" But not so fast; natural gas companies add that distinctive (and for most of us, distinctly unpleasant) odor to their colorless, odorless, tasteless, and highly flammable product, so that we'll know it's there. If there's a gas leak of any substantial amount, we can smell it—so as you can see, the primitive senses protect us still. Loss of the ability to detect the odor could prove deadly if you unwittingly strike a match where natural gas has leaked and accumulated. A danger to be sure, but even more important, the loss of the sense of smell can be an outward sign of a struggling brain; it can even predict greater risk for developing Alzheimer's disease. This has been documented by the University of Pennsylvania Smell Identification Test (UPSIT). See pages 212–213.

Alzheimer's Disease: The Thief of Memory

This is not specifically a book about Alzheimer's disease, but because this condition represents the single most devastating cause for memory impairment, no book on memory would be complete without its inclusion. Dr. Alois Alzheimer first described the disease that bears his name 100 years ago, and yet it's certain cause and cure still elude us. That's not to say a century of scientific examination has been for naught; we know a tremendous amount about the development of the disease all the way to the microscopic and molecular levels. Ongoing research may unlock the secrets to what causes it, and a number of medications currently on the market have proven modestly helpful in lessening its symptoms; others under development may hold the key to preventing its devastation in the future. But apart from medications, there is reason for hope and here's why.

One hot bed of research centers on the brain's ability to metabolize glucose (blood sugar) properly. Scientists have used a specialized method of imaging the brain, called positron emission tomography (PET), that can detect and quantify the ability of different regions of the brain to burn glucose. PET scanning has uncovered an important clue: the earliest finding in Alzheimer's disease is a subtle decrease in brain glucose metabolism, particularly in the areas most closely tied to memory. Among people who carry the apolipoprotein E (APOE) epsilon 4 (ϵ4) gene, which puts them at high risk for later developing Alzheimer's disease, such scans can identify changes in glucose metabolism almost 40 years before memory starts to fail.

Animal research confirms the connection between abnormal sugar metabolism and the development of Alzheimer's disease. In laboratory experiments, researchers can artificially disrupt blood sugar and insulin metabolism in a variety of ways. When they do, the test animals almost instantly develop a severe form of insulin resistance, lose their memory functions, and become quite demented. It is interesting that these animals also develop deposits in their brains that have a striking resemblance to the changes seen in the brains of humans with Alzheimer's disease. Although that connection is intriguing, the degree of instant insulin resistance that occurs in this experimental setting isn't what happens in humans who become insulin resistant and diabetic over the course of many years.

To more closely mimic the human situation, researchers created a version of diabetes and insulin resistance in lab mice by feeding them a diet containing added fructose, a simple sugar found naturally in limited amounts in fruit (hence its name) and in big amounts in high-fructose corn syrup, the sweetener used in nondiet colas and in most commercially prepared candies and other sweet treats. When fed this diet, the mice (like their human counterparts) gradually become insulin resistant and ultimately develop diabetes. Even in this more gradual scenario, however, the mice responded in a similar fashion, losing memory, developing brain deposits, and becoming demented.

Coupled with human PET scan studies demonstrating early abnormalities in glucose metabolism in the memory-sensitive areas of the brains of people carrying the APOE ε4 gene, this research suggests a fundamental link between normal glucose metabolism and brain health (or conversely, a relationship between abnormal glucose metabolism and brain disease). That people with diabetes, glucose intolerance, and varying degrees of insulin resistance (even in the face of normal blood sugar) are at double the risk of developing memory impairment further implicates the glucose-insulin system as a major player in determining how well memory is preserved as we age. Why might this be?

TANGLING THE MIND

The brains of patients with Alzheimer's disease develop a characteristic microscopic finding: clumps of protein—called neurofibrillary tangles—that are deposited inside the brain cells long before symptoms of their disease become apparent. First seen in and around the memory centers, the tangles spread in a predictable fashion throughout the brain and represent the only visible finding that correlates with the extent and severity of Alzheimer's symptoms—that is, the more numerous and dense the tangles, the worse the symptoms.

What are the tangles? You'll recall from Chapter 2 that the formation of synapses, the interconnections between brain cells, occurs somewhat like raising a circus tent—with a floppy canvas dome (the cell membrane) supported by tent poles (microfilaments) lashed together with ropes (tau proteins). The cells coordinate the attachment of the tau proteins to the microfilaments through a biochemical process called phosphorylation, which you can think of as the production of strong glue that allows the poles to stick together securely. Without enough glue, the poles come loose; too much of it and everything sticks together in a knotted mess, which is pretty much what happens when tangles are formed. They develop because of excess or unrestrained phosphorylation of tau proteins in a process called hyperphosphorylation.

Because of their almost universal presence in patients with this disease and their intimate relationship with symptom severity, these tangles have become the focus of an enormous amount of research. And, as is so often the case in medicine, help appeared from a most unlikely place: hibernating ground squirrels.

When ground squirrels hibernate in winter, their body temperature falls, their metabolic processes slow dramatically, and their brain activity becomes almost nonexistent. As the weather warms, the animals emerge from their torpor. During this warming transition, their memory functions remain somewhat impaired; but once they attain normal body temperature, their brain function returns completely. Hibernation, it seems, represents a fully reversible process for body and brain in the ground squirrel, prompting researchers looking for answers in Alzheimer's disease to study the changes that take place in the squirrels' brains during the process. What they've found is truly amazing.

During the period of suspended animation, structures somewhat akin to tangles temporarily appear in the squirrels' brains, but they then regress—

unlike in Alzheimer's disease, in which they appear and remain permanently. The big question researchers want to answer is what makes the squirrels' tangles regress, because understanding this phenomenon could perhaps unlock the mysteries of why they persist in the human brain and how to reverse that process. In squirrels, at least, it seems to be related to temperature.

Although it would seem logical that once a ground squirrel attained a deep level of hibernation, it would remain in that energy-conserving state until the spring thaw, but that is not the case. Hibernating animals go through cyclic periods of arousal during which they partially warm up, increasing both their metabolic rate and their brain wave activity. Because of the tremendous energy cost of these episodes of arousal, scientists believe they must play an important role in the hibernation process but as yet haven't definitively proven how.

What is known is that there is a reduction in or lowering of the phosphorylation state of the tau proteins during these arousal periods, which scientists believe to be a pivotal event in preventing the phenomenon that turns normal tau proteins into tangles. It appears that the squirrel brain is programmed to warm just enough and to alter the phosphorylation process just enough to keep its synaptic interconnections strong and preserve its memory functions during the hibernation period without going too far. Without the programmed partial rewarming cycles—that is, with prolonged, continuous chilling and brain inactivity—there would be a wholesale loss of brain cell connections during hibernation that would require relearning of a veritable universe (at least in squirrel terms) of important information upon reawakening. Perhaps without the cycling, the tangles would even become permanent.

It's back to the Goldilocks principles: The amount of phosphorylation needs to be just right in both degree and duration. Prolonged periods of excess phosphorylation produce the brain equivalent of powerful glue, the deposition of tangles, and the consequent destruction of brain cells and memory. But humans aren't ground squirrels and we don't hibernate. So what's all this got to do with us?

The crucial link that connects brain glucose metabolism, synapse preservation, tau proteins, and tangles in humans appears to be the prevailing level of insulin resistance in the brain; because, like temperature in the squirrels, insulin has the ability to regulate the degree and duration of phosphorylation in humans. So close is this link that researchers at Brown University in Rhode Island even coined the phrase type 3 diabetes to describe what develops in the brains of people with Alzheimer's disease. The implication is that if insulin resistance in the brain becomes a permanent condition, it will tend to produce more intense and prolonged degrees of tau hyperphosphorylation (more glue) and thereby increase the development of the tangles, which are intimately linked with the dementia of Alzheimer's.

To compound the problem further, the insulin-resistant brain, like the insulin-resistant body, cannot properly use glucose, which immediately deprives the brain cells of adequate fuel for energy. (Recall that the PET scan images of the brains of individuals at high risk of developing Alzheimer's disease showed this very defect present decades before their symptoms appeared.) When glucose metabolism falters, energy supplies run short, the brain cells suffer functional brown outs, cell to cell connections degenerate, and brain fog ensues. Without sufficient energy, the cell will be unable to control the inflow of excitatory molecules, such as calcium, into its interior. If this condition is left uncorrected, the brain cell will die.

How can the process be reversed? This may be achieved by correcting insulin resistance in the body and the brain through proper nutrition, added nutrients, and lifestyle changes as outlined in Chapters 4, 5, and 6. Controlling the first defect—that of developing abnormal glucose metabolism in the brain—offers the best hope for preventing the development of Alzheimer's disease in those at high risk and to potentially stabilize brain function in those for whom memory impairment has begun. The insulin-resistant brain must have alternative fuels to glucose to burn, such as the ketone bodies naturally produced on the ketogenic diet and supported by regularly taking the Ketogenic Cocktail (page 203) and the Anti-Excitatory Cocktail (page 204). Giving the brain cells alternative fuels, such as ketones, to burn in the face of a glucose shortage sounds promising, but does it really work? An ingenious experiment suggests it does.

KETONES TO THE RESCUE

To investigate whether ketones could substitute for glucose as a brain fuel, researchers gave study volunteers a dose of insulin through an intravenous (IV) line in an amount calculated to drop their blood sugar to a level low enough to deprive the brain of glucose. As expected, the sudden drop in blood sugar caused the subjects to develop symptoms: nausea, lightheadedness, dizziness, and confusion. The researchers then repeated the experiment, but gave one group of volunteers a dose of ketones in their IV lines before giving the insulin. Just as before, the blood sugar fell to low levels in all subjects, but the group who received the ketones did not develop symptoms of low blood sugar; they acted and thought normally, proving that energy generated in the brain by ketones can substitute perfectly for the loss of glucose.

Can ketones help the brains of people with impaired glucose metabolism, such as those with the APOE ε4 gene, those with mild cognitive impairment, and those with frank Alzheimer's disease—not in the research lab, but in the real world? Yes, it appears they can! In another study, researchers gave a group of patients with Alzheimer's disease supplemental MCT oil (a component of my Ketogenic Cocktail) and noted improvements in both memory and ability to think, reason, and focus—without drugs or their severe side effects.

Just as with migraines, hot flashes, and the brain fog of menopause, my experience has taught me that when good brains go bad, no matter what the cause—trauma, disease, age, disuse, or abuse—good nutrition can be the cornerstone to strengthen the struggling brain and restore its proper function, giving us all greater hope for a brighter future.

That future begins now as you begin to incorporate the nutrition and exercise principles into your daily life. Remember that nutritional changes aren't fast acting like a dose of aspirin. Rather, they occur gradually over a period of weeks and months as bit by bit you replace poor-quality fats with good ones; replenish stores of brain-critical nutrients to appropriate levels; increase muscle, bone, and brain mass; and form new cellular connections. Work all components of the Brain Trust Program diligently, be patient, be persistent, and you will reap the rewards of quicker thought processing and reflexes, a sharper memory, better focus, improved sleep, and a happier mood. All from building a stronger, healthier brain. When you do, I'd love to hear about it; contact me at www.drmccleary.com.

RESOURCES

RECOMMENDED READING AND VIEWING

Ross Pelton, James B. LaValle, Ernest B. Hawkins, and Daniel Krinsky. *Drug-Induced Nutrient Depletion Handbook*. Lexi-Comp, Hudson, OH (2001). This text contains information on nutrients that can be depleted by pharmaceuticals.

The Secret Life of the Brain. Produced by David Grubin, 2002. This PBS series offers a history of the brain, its anatomy, and physical development from childhood through adult life. The series is available on VHS and DVD through the PBS website (www.pbs.org).

WEBSITES OF HELPFUL ORGANIZATIONS AND INSTITUTIONS

National Institute of Neurological Disorders and Stroke. "Brain Basics: Know Your Brain." Available at www.ninds.nih.gov/disorders/brain_basics/know_your_brain.htm. At this site you'll find a primer on the brain and brain anatomy for nonscientists.

U.S. National Library of Medicine, National Institutes of Health. Available at www.nlm.nih.gov. This site provides access to the world's largest medical library.

The National Association for Health & Fitness and the California Governor's Council on Physical Fitness & Sports. Available at www.physicalfitness.org.

The Better Hearing Institute. Available at www.betterhearing.org. This organization is dedicated to helping people with hearing loss.

The American Association for Geriatric Psychiatry. Available at www.aagpgpa.org. This association is for doctors who specialize in caring for the mental health of older persons. The website contains information on a broad array of mental health issues.

The National Sleep Foundation. Available at www.sleepfoundation.org. This site lists the names of sleep specialists, contains information on sleep disorders, and offers educational publications.

The American Academy of Ophthalmology. Available at www.eyenet.org. This site provides information about numerous eye disorders and other causes of vision loss.

The American Diabetes Association. Available at www.diabetes.org. This association helps you find information about diabetes, diabetic complications, and other related issues.

The American Parkinson Disease Association. Available at www.apdaparkin son.org. This site contains educational material on Parkinson's disease and referrals for specialists and community services.

The Alzheimer's Association. Available at www.alz.org. This site provides information on clinical trials and links to many other related sites.

The American Brain Tumor Association. Available at www.abta.org. This site provides in-depth information of all sorts about brain cancers and includes links to various helpful sites about everything to do with brain tumors.

Brains.org. Available at www.brains.org. This site provides information to people involved in education and parenting.

The Brain Injury Association. Available at www.biausa.org. The mission of this association is to create a better future through brain injury awareness, prevention, research, education, and advocacy.

BrainBashers. Available at www.brainbashers.com. An online resource for brainteasers, puzzles, online games, optical illusions, and jigsaw puzzles.

RECOMMENDED SOURCES OF NUTRITIONAL SUPPLEMENTS AND ORGANIC, FREE-RANGE, AND UNIQUE FOODS

Advanced Metabolic Research Group. Available at www.lucidal.com. This site contains details about Lucidal, the clinically tested nutritional supplement for the brain that I developed and patented.

Omega Natural Sceince. Available at www.omegabrite.com. This site offers information about OmegaBrite, one of the best long-chain omega-3 fatty acid supplements around; developed and researched by a Harvard physician. Each OmegaBrite capsule is manufactured to ensure the highest quality by distillation for purity and processing in a nitrogen environment.

Eagle Eye Wine. Available at www.eagleeyewine.com. This site provides information about organic Eagle Eye Wine, grown in Napa, California.

LocalHarvest. Available at www.localharvest.org. This site provides links to purveyors of organic produce near your home.

Broken Arrow Ranch. Available at www.brokenarrowranch.com. Learn more about free-range meat products produced in Ingram, Texas.

Woodstock Water Buffalo Co. Available at www.woodstockwaterbuffalo.com. Browse this site to learn about the virtues and health benefits of water buffalo milk, cheese, and yogurt produced in South Woodstock, Vermont.

Neptune Technologies & Bioresources Inc. Available at www.neptunebiotech .com. Here you can learn more about krill oil and its importance to your brain. *Note:* Krill oil is available at my website (www.drmccleary.com) or from my colleagues' website (www.proteinpower.com).

BIBLIOGRAPHY

GENERAL

Andrews, M. H., and S. G. Matthews. "Antenatal Glucocorticoids: Is There Cause for Concern?" *Fetal and Maternal Medicine Review* 14 (2003): 329–354.

Arendt, T., M. K. Bruckner, H. J. Gertz, and N. Marcova. "Cortical Distribution of Neurofibrillary Tangles in Alzheimer's Disease Matches the Pattern of Neurons That Retain Their Capacity of Plastic Remodeling in the Adult Brain." *Neuroscience* 83 (1998): 991–1002.

Arendt, T. "Alzheimer's Disease as a Disorder of Mechanisms Underlying Structural Brain Self-Organization." *Neuroscience* 102 (2001): 723–765.

Arendt, T. "Disturbance of Neuronal Plasticity Is a Critical Pathogenetic Event in Alzheimer's Disease." *International Journal of Developmental Neuroscience* 19 (2001): 231–245.

Arendt, T. "Neurodegeneration and Plasticity." *International Journal of Developmental Neuroscience* 22 (2004): 507–514.

Barrett, A. M., P. J. Eslinger, N. H. Ballentine, and K. M. Heilman. "Unawareness of Cognitive Deficit (Cognitive Anosognosia) in Probable AD and Control Subjects." *Neurology* 64 (2005): 693–699.

Brookmeyer, R., S. Gray, and C. Kawas. "Projections of Alzheimer's Disease in the United States and the Public Health Impact of Delaying Disease Onset." *American Journal of Public Health* 88 (1998): 1337–1342.

Choi, D. W. "Glutamate, Cell Death, and Hats Off to Carl Cotman." *Neurochemical Research* 28 (2003): 1621–1624.

Den Heijer, T., L. J. Launer, N. D. Prins, E. J. van Dijk, S. E. Vermeer, A. Hofman, P. J. Koudstaal, and M.M.B. Breteler. "Association Between Blood Pressure, White Matter Lesions and Atrophy of the Medial Temporal Lobe." *Neurology* 64 (2005): 263–267.

Fossati, P., A. Radtchenko, and P. Boyer. "Neuroplasticity: From MRI to Depressive Symptoms." *European Neuropsychopharmacol* 14 (2004): S503–S510.

Gianaros, P. J., P. J. Greer, C. M. Ryan, and J. R. Jennings. "Higher Blood Pressure Predicts Lower Regional Grey Matter Volume: Consequences on Short-Term Information Processing." *NeuroImage* 31 (2006): 754–765.

Gold, S. M., I. Dziobek, K. Rogers, A. Bayoumy, P. F. McHugh, and A. Convit. "Hypertension and Hypothalamo-Pituitary-Adrenal Axis Hyperactivity Affect Frontal Lobe Integrity." *Journal of Clinical Endocrinology and Metabolism* 90 (2005): 3262–3267.

Grady, C. L., M. V. Springer, D. Honggwanishkul, A. R. McIntosh, and G. Winocur. "Age-Related Changes in Brain Activity Across the Adult Lifespan." *Journal of Cognitive Neuroscience* 18 (2006): 227–241.

Heflin, L. H., B. E. Meyerowitz, P. Hall, P. Lichtenstein, B. Johansson, N. L. Pedersen, and M. Gatz. "Cancer as a Risk Factor for Long-Term Cognitive Deficits and Dementia." *Jounral of the National Cancer Institute* 97 (2005): 854–856.

Huang, Y. "Apolipoprotein E and Alzheimer Disease." *Neurology* 66, suppl. 1 (2006): S79–S85.

Hynd, M. R., H. L. Scott, and P. R. Dodd. "Glutamate-Mediated Excitotoxicity and Neurodegeneration in Alzheimer's Disease." *Neurochemistry International* 45 (2004): 583–595.

Ikonomovic, M. D., K. Uryu, E. E. Abrahamson, J. R. Ciallella, J. Q. Trojanowski, V.M.Y. Lee, R. S. Clark, D. W. Marion, S. R. Wisniewski, and S. T. DeKosky. "Alzheimer's Pathology in Human Temporal Cortex Surgically Excised After Severe Brain Injury." *Experiment Neurology* 190 (2004): 192–203.

Kapoor, A., E. Dunn, A. Kostacki, M. H. Andrews, and S. G. Matthews. "Fetal Programming of Hypothalamo-Pituitary-Adrenal Function: Prenatal Stress and Glucocorticoids." *Journal of Physiology* 572 (2006): 31–44.

Kawashima, R., K. Okita, R. Yamazaki, N. Tajima, H. Yoshida, M. Taira, K. Iwata, T. Sasaki, K. Maeyama, N. Usui, and K. Sugimoto. "Reading Aloud and Arithmetic Calculation Improve Frontal Function of People with Dementia." *Journal of Gerontology, Series A, Biological Sciences and Medical Sciences* 60 (2005): 380–384.

Kidd, P. M. "Neurodegeneration from Mitochondrial Insufficiency: Nutrients, Stem Cells, Growth Factors and Prospects for Brain Rebuilding Using Integrative Management." *Alternative Medicine Review* 10 (2005): 268–290.

Luchsinger, J. A., C. Reitz, L. S. Honig, M. X. Tang, S. Shea, and R. Mayeux. "Aggregation of Vascular Risk Factors and Risk of Alzheimer Disease." *Neurology* 65 (2005): 545–551.

Lupien, S. J., and M. Lepage. "Stress, Memory and the Hippocampus: Can't Live With It, Can't Live Without It." *Behavioral Brain Research* 127 (2001): 137–158.

Lye, T. C., and E. A. Shores. "Traumatic Brain Injury as a Risk Factor for Alzheimer's Disease: A Review." *Neuropsychology Review* 10 (2000): 115–129.

Mesulam, M. M. "Neuroplasticity Failure in Alzheimer's Disease: Bridging the Gap Between Plaques and Tangles." *Neuron* 24 (1999): 521–529.

Montaran, M. F., E. Drapeau, D. Dupret, P. Kitchener, C. Aurousseau, M. Le Moal, P. V. Piazza, and D. N. Abrous. "Lifelong Corticosterone Level Determines Age-Related Decline in Neurogenesis and Memory." *Neurobiology of Aging* 27 (2006): 645–654.

Mortimer, J. A., D. A. Snowdon, and W. R. Markesbery. "Head Circumference, Education and Risk of Dementia: Findings from the Nun Study." *Journal of Clinical and Experimental Neuropsychology* 25 (2003): 671–679.

Mukamal, K. J., L. H. Kuller, A. L. Fitzpatrick, W. T. Longstreth Jr., M. A. Mittleman, and D. S. Siscovick. "Prospective Study of Alcohol Consumption and Risk of Dementia in Older Adults." *Journal of the American Medical Association* 289 (2003): 1405–1413.

Nathanielcz, P. W., and V. Padmanabhan. "Developmental Origin of Health and Disease." *Journal of Physiology* 572 (2006): 3–4.

Otto, M., S. Holthusen, E. Bahn, N. Sohnchen, J. Wiltfang, R. Geese, A. Fischer, and C. D. Reimers. "Boxing and Running Lead to a Rise in Serum Levels of S-100B Protein." *International Journal of Sports Medicine* 21 (2000): 551–555.

Phillips, D.I.W., and A. Jones. "Fetal Programming of Autonomic and HPA Function: Do People Who Were Small Babies Have Enhanced Stress Responses?" *Journal of Physiology* 572 (2006): 45–50.

Radley, J. J., and J. H. Morrison. "Repeated Stress and Structural Plasticity in the Brain." *Ageing Research Review* 4 (2005): 271–287.

Richards, M., and I. J. Deary. "A Life Course Approach to Cognitive Reserve: A Model for Cognitive Aging and Development." *Annals of Neurology* 58 (2005): 617–622.

Riley, K. P., D. A. Snowdon, M. F. Desrosiers, and W. R. Markesbery. "Early Life Linguistic Ability, Late Life Cognitive Function and Neuropathology: Findings from the Nun Study." *Neurobiology of Aging* 26 (2005): 341–347.

Scarmeas, N., E. Zarahn, K. E. Anderson, J. Hilton, J. Flynn, R. L. Van Heertum, H. A. Sackeim, and Y. Stern. "Cognitive Reserve Modulates Functional Brain Responses During Memory Tasks: A PET Study in Healthy Young and Elderly Subjects." *NeuroImage* 19 (2003): 1215–1227.

Sundstrom, A., P. Marklund, L. G. Nilsson, M. Cruts, R. Adolfsson, C. Van Broeckhoven, and L. Nyberg. "APOE Influences on Neuropsychological Function After Mild Head Injury." *Neurology* 62 (2004): 1963–1966.

Van Osch, L.A.D.M., E. Hogervorst, M. Combrinck, and A. D. Smith. "Low Thyroid-Stimulating Hormone as an Independent Risk Factor for Alzheimer Disease." *Neurology* 62 (2004): 1967–1971.

Whalley, L. J., I. J. Deary, C. L. Appleton, and J. M. Starr. "Cognitive Reserve and the Neurobiology of Cognitive Aging." *Ageing Research Review* 3 (2004): 369–382.

Whitmer, R. A., S. Sidney, J. Selby, S. C. Johnston, and K. Yaffe. "Midlife Cardiovascular Risk Factors and Risk of Dementia in Late Life." *Neurology* 64 (2005): 277–281.

Wolf, H., A. Hensel, T. Arendt, M. Kivipelto, B. Winblad, and H. J. Gertz. "Serum Lipids and Hippocampal Volume: The Link to Alzheimer's Disease?" *Annals of Neurology* 56 (2004): 745–749.

INFORMATION ON NUTRIENTS AND NUTRITIONAL SUPPLEMENTS

Albrecht, J., and A. Schousboe. "Taurine Interaction with Neurotransmitter Receptors in the CNS: An Update." *Neurochemistry Research* 30 (2005): 1615–1621.

Andress, R. H., A. D. Ducray, A. W. Huber, A. Perez-Bouza, S. H. Krebs, U. Schlattner, R. W. Seiler, T. Wallimann, and H. R. Widmer. "Effects of Creatine Treatment on Survival and Differentiation of GABA-ergic Neurons in Cultured Striatal Tissue." *Journal of Neurochemistry* 95 (2005): 33–45.

Bastianetto, S., Z. X. Yao, V. Papadopoulos, and R. Quirion. "Neuroprotective Effects of Green and Black Teas and Their Catechin Esters Against Beta-Amyloid-Induced Toxicity." *European Journal of Neuroscience* 23 (2006): 55–64.

Bonoczk, P., B. Gulyas, V. Adam-Vizi, A. Nemes, E. Karpati, B. Kiss, M. Kapas, C. Szantay, I. Koncz, T. Zelles, and A. Vas. "Role of Sodium Channel Inhibition in Neuroprotection: Effect of Vinpocetine." *Brain Research Bulletin* 53 (2000): 245–254.

Bottiglieri, T., and R. Diaz-Arrastia. "Hyperhomocysteinemia and Cognitive Function: More than Just a Casual Link?" *American Journal of Clinical Nutrition* 82 (2005): 493–494.

Cohn, J. S. "Oxidized Fat in the Diet, Postprandial Lipaemia and Cardiovascular Disease." *Current Opinion in Lipidology* 13 (2002): 19–24.

Cole, G. M., G. P. Lim, F. Yang, B. Teter, A. Begum, Q. Ma, M. E. Harris-White, and S. A. Frautschy. "Prevention of Alzheimer's Disease: Omega-3 Fatty Acid and Phenolic Anti-Oxidant Interventions." *Neurobiology of Aging* 26, suppl. 1 (2005): 133–136.

El Idrissi, A., and E. Trenkner. "Growth Factors and Taurine Protect Against Excitotoxicity by Stabilizing Calcium Homeostasis and Energy Metabolism." *Journal of Neuroscience* 19 (1999): 9459–9468.

Foley, D. J., and L. R. White. "Dietary Intake of Antioxidants and Risk of Alzheimer Disease." *Journal of the American Medical Association* 287 (2002): 3261–3263.

Friedland, R. P. "Fish Consumption and the Risk of Alzheimer Disease." *Archives of Neurology* 60 (2003): 923–924.

Galli, R. L., D. F. Bielinski, A. Szprengiel, B. Shukitt-Hale, and J. A. Joseph. "Blueberry Supplemented Diet Reverses Age-Related Decline in Hippocampal HS70 Neuroprotection." *Neurobiology of Aging* 27 (2006): 344–350.

Gordon, P. K., S. V. Nigam, J. A. Weitz, J. R. Dave, B. P. Doctor, and H. S. Ved. "The NMDA Receptor Ion Channel: Site for Binding of Huperzine A." *Journal of Applied Toxicology* 21 (2001): S47–S51.

Held, K., I. A. Antonijevic, H. Kunzel, M. Uhr, T. C. Wetter, I. C. Golly, A. Steiger, and H. Murck. "Oral Mg++ Supplementation Reverses Age-Related Neuroendocrine and Sleep EEG Changes in Humans." *Pharmacopsychiatry* 35 (2002): 135–143.

Joseph, J. A., N. A. Denisova, G. Arendash, M. Gordon, D. Diamond, B. Shukitt-Hale, and D. Morgan. "Blueberry Supplementation Enhances Signaling and Prevents Behavioral Deficits in an Alzheimer Disease Model." *Nutritional Neuroscience* 6 (2003): 153–162.

Joseph, J. A., B. Shukitt-Hale, and G. Casadesus. "Reversing the Deleterious Effects of Aging on Neuronal Communication and Behavior: Beneficial Properties of Fruit Polyphenolic Compounds." *American Journal of Clinical Nutrition* 81, suppl. (2005): 313S–316S.

Kruman, I. I., P. R. Mouton, R. Emokpae Jr., R. G. Cutler, and M. P. Mattson. "Folate Deficiency Inhibits Proliferation of Adult Hippocampal Progenitors." *Neuroreport* 16 (2005): 1055–1059.

Kuriyama, S., A. Hozawa, K. Ohmori, T. Shimazu, T. Matsui, S. Ebihara, S. Awata, R. Nagatomi, H. Arai, I. Tsuli. "Green Tea Consumption and Cognitive Function: A Cross-Sectional Study from the Tsurugaya Project." *American Journal of Clinical Nutrition* 83 (2006): 355–361.

Lau, F. C., B. Shukitt-Hale, and J. A. Joseph. "The Beneficial Effects of Fruit Polyphenols on Brain Aging." *Neurobiology of Aging* 26, suppl. 1 (2005): 128–132.

Lonergan, P. E., D.S.D. Martin, D. F. Horrobin, and M. A. Lynch. "Neuroprotective Actions of Eicosapentaenoic Acid on Lipopolysaccharide-Induced Dysfunction in Rat Hippocampus." *Journal of Neurochemistry* 91 (2004): 20–29.

Louzada, P. R., A.C.P. Lima, D. L. Mendonca-Silva, F. Noel, F. G. De Mello, and S. T. Ferreira. "Taurine Prevents the Neurotoxicity of β-Amyloid and Glutamate Receptor Agonists: Activation of GABA Receptors and Possible Implications for Alzheimer's Disease and Other Neurological Disorders." *FASEB Journal* 18 (2004): 511–518.

Molnar, P., and S. L. Erdo. "Vinpocetine is as Potent as Dilantin to Block Voltage-Gated Na+ Channels in Rat Cortical Neurons." *European Journal of Pharmacology* 6 (1995): 303–306.

Moore, M. E., A. Piazza, Y. McCartney, and M. A. Lynch. "Evidence that Vitamin D Reverses the Age-Related Inflammatory Changes in the Rat Hippocampus." *Biochemistry Society Transactions* 33 (2005): 577.

Morris, M. C., D. A. Evans, J. L. Bienias, P. A. Scherr, C. C. Tangney, L. E. Hebert, D. A. Bennett, R. S. Wilson, and N. Aggarwal. "Dietary Niacin and the Risk of Incident Alzheimer's Disease and of Cognitive Decline." *Journal of Neurology, Neurosurgery and Psychiatry* 75 (2004): 1093–1099.

Morris, M. C., D. A. Evans, J. L. Bienias, C. C. Tangney, D. A. Bennett, R. S. Wilson, N. Aggarwal, and J. Schneider. "Consumption of Fish and N-3 Fatty Acids and Risk of Incident Alzheimer Disease." *Archives of Neurology* 60 (2003): 940–946.

Morris, M. C., D. A. Evans, C. C. Tangney, J. L. Bienias, and R. S. Wilson. "Fish Consumption and Cognitive Decline with Age in a Large Community Study." *Archives of Neurology* 62 (2005): 1849–1853.

Paula-Lima, A. C., F. G. De Felice, J. Brito-Moreira, and S. T. Ferriera. "Activation of GABA (A) Receptors by Taurine and Muscimol Blocks the Neurotoxicity of β-Amyloid in Rat Hippocampal and Cortical Neurons." *Neuropharmacology* 49 (2005): 1140–1148.

Quadri, P., C. Fragiacomo, R. Pezzati, E. Zanda, G. Forloni, M. Tettamanti, and U. Lucca. "Homocysteine, Folate and Vitamin B-12 in Mild Cognitive Impairment, Alzheimer Disease and Vascular Dementia." *American Journal of Clinical Nutrition* 80 (2004): 114–122.

Quinn, J. F., J. R. Bussiere, R. S. Hammond, T. J. Montine, E. Henson, R. E. Jones, and R. W. Stackman Jr. "Chronic Dietary Alpha-Lipoic Acid Reduces Deficits in Hippocampal Memory of Aged Tg2576 Mice." *Neurobiology of Aging* (forthcoming).

Ravaglia, G., P. Forti, F. Maioli, M. Martelli, L. Servadei, N. Brunetti, E. Porcellini, and F. Licastro. "Homocysteine and Folate as Risk Factors for Dementia and Alzheimer Disease." *American Journal of Clinical Nutrition* 82 (2005): 636–643.

Shishodia, S., G. Sethi, and B. A. Aggarwal. "Curcumin: Getting Back to the Roots." *Annals of the New York Academy of Science* 1056 (2005): 206–217.

Tucker, K. L., N. Qiao, T. Scott, I. Rosenberg, and A. Spiro III. "High Homocysteine and Low B Vitamins Predict Cognitive Decline in Aging Men: The Veterans Affairs Normative Aging Study." *American Journal of Clinical Nutrition* 82 (2005): 627–635.

Wang, R., and X. C. Tang. "Neuroprotective Effects of Huperzine A: A Natural Cholinesterase Inhibitor for the Treatment of Alzheimer's Disease." *Neurosignals* 14 (2005): 71–82.

Wu, A., Z. Ying, and F. Gomez-Pinilla. "Dietary Omega-3 Fatty Acids Normalize BDNF Levels, Reduce Oxidative Damage, and Counteract Learning Disability After Traumatic Brain Injury in Rats." *Journal of Neurotrauma* 21 (2004): 1457–1467.

Wu, H., Y. Jin, J. Wei, H. Jin, D. Sha, and J. Y. Wu. "Mode of Action of Taurine as a Neuroprotector." *Brain Research* 1038 (2005): 123–131.

Yehuda, S., S. Rabinovitz, and D. I. Mostofsky. "Essential Fatty Acids and the Brain: From Infancy to Aging." *Neurobiology of Aging* 26, suppl. 1 (2005): 98–102.

Yehuda, S. "Omega-6/Omega-3 Ratio and Brain-Related Functions." *World Review of Nutrition and Dietetics* 92 (2003): 37–56.

Youdim, K. A., B. Shukitt-Hale, and J. A. Joseph. "Flavonoids and the Brain: Interactions at the Blood-Brain Barrier and Their Physiological Effects on the

Central Nervous System." *Free Radical Biology & Medicine* 37 (2004): 1683–1693.

Zandi, P. P., J. C. Anthony, A. S. Khachaturian, S. V. Stone, D. Gustafson, J. T. Tschanz, M. C. Norton, K. A. Welsh-Bohmer, and J.C.S. Breitner (for the Cache County Study Group). "Reduced Risk of Alzheimer Disease in Users of Antioxidant Vitamin Supplements." *Archives of Neurology* 61 (2004): 82–88.

Zangara, A. "The Psychopharmacology of Huperzine A: An Alkaloid with Cognitive Enhancing and Neuroprotective Properties of Interest in the Treatment of Alzheimer's Disease." *Pharmacology, Biochemistry and Behavior* 75 (2003): 675–686.

Zelles, T., L. Franklin, I. Koncz, B. Lendvai, and G. Zsilla. "The Nootropic Drug Vinpocetine Inhibits Veratridine-Induced [Ca+]i Increase in Rat Hippocampal CA1 Pyramidal Cells." *Neurochemistry Research* 26 (2001): 1095–1100.

Zhao, P., Y. L. Huang, and J. S. Cheng. "Taurine Antagonizes Calcium Overload Induced by Glutamate or Chemical Hypoxia in Cultured Rat Hippocampal Neurons." *Neuroscience Letters* 268 (1999): 25–28.

INFORMATION ON HEARING AND TINNITUS

Attias, J., S. Sapir, I. Bresloff, I. Reshaf-Haran, and H. Ising. "Reduction in Noise-Induced Temporary Threshold Shift in Humans Following Oral Magnesium Intake." *Clinical Otolaryngology and Allied Sciences* 29 (2004): 635–641.

Attias, J., G. Weisz, S. Almog, A. Shahar, M. Wiener, Z. Joachims, A. Netzer, H. Ising, E. Rebentisch, and T. Guenther. "Oral Magnesium Intake Reduces Permanent Hearing Loss Induced by Noise Exposure." *American Journal of Otolaryngology* 15 (1994): 26–32.

Cevette, M. J., J. Vormann, and K. Franz. "Magnesium and Hearing." *Journal of the American Academy of Audiology* 14 (2003): 202–212.

Eggermont, J. J. "Tinnitus: Neurobiological Substrates." *Drug Discovery Today* 10 (2005): 1283–1290.

Gathwala, G. "Neuronal Protection with Magnesium." *Indian Journal of Pediatrics* 68 (2001): 417–419.

Haupt, H., and F. Scheibe. "Preventive Magnesium Supplement Protects the Inner Ear Against Noise-Induced Impairment of Blood Flow and Oxygenation in the Guinea Pig." *Magnesium Research* 15 (2002): 17–25.

Joachims, Z., A. Netzer, H. Ising, E. Rebentisch, J. Attias, and T. Gunther. "Oral

Magnesium Supplementation as Prophylaxis for Noise-Induced Hearing Loss: Results of a Double Blind Field Study." *Schriftenr Ver Wasser Boden Lufthyg* 88 (1993): 503–516.

Kaltenbach, J. A., J. Zhang, and P. Finlayson. "Tinnitus as a Plastic Phenomenon and Its Possible Neural Underpinnings in the Dorsal Cochlear Nucleus." *Hearing Research* 206 (2005): 200–226.

Lynch, E. D., and J. Kil. "Compounds for the Prevention and Treatment of Noise-Induced Hearing Loss." *Drug Discovery Today* 10 (2005): 1291–1298.

Moller, A. R. "Symptoms and Signs Caused by Neural Plasticity." *Neurology Research* 23 (2001): 565–572.

Oestreicher, E., W. Arnold, K. Ehrenberger, and D. Felix. "Memantine Suppresses the Glutaminergic Neurotransmission of Mammalian Inner Hair Cells." *ORL, Journal for Oto-Rhino-Laryngology and Its Relative Specialties* 60 (1998): 18–21.

Oestreicher, E., W. Arnold, K. Ehrenberger, and D. Felix. "New Approaches for Inner Ear Therapy with Glutamate Antagonists." *Acta Oto-Laryngologica* 119 (1999): 174–178.

Oestreicher, E., A. Wolfgang, and D. Felix. "Neurotransmission of the Cochlear Inner Hair Cell Synapse—Implications for Inner Ear Therapy." *Advances in Otorhinolaryngology* 59 (2002): 131–139.

Puel, J. L., J. Ruel, G. d'Aldin, and R. Pujol. "Excitotoxicity and Repair of Cochlear Synapses After Noise-Trauma Induced Hearing Loss." *Neuroreport* 9 (1998): 2109–2114.

Pujol, R., G. Rebillard, J. L. Puel, M. Lenoir, M. Eybalin, and M. Recasens. "Glutamate Neurotoxicity in the Cochlea: A Possible Consequence of Ischemic or Anoxic Conditions Occurring in Ageing." *Acta Oto-Laryngologica Supplementum* 476 (1990): 32–36.

Salvi, R. J., J. Wang, and D. Ding. "Auditory Plasticity and Hyperactivity Following Cochlear Damage." *Hearing Research* 147 (2000): 261–274.

Scheibe, F., H. Haupt, and H. Ising. "Preventive Effect of Magnesium Supplement on Noise-Induced Hearing Loss in the Guinea Pig." *European Archives of Otorhinolaryngology* 257 (2000): 10–16.

Seidman, M. D., N. Ahmad, and U. Bai. "Molecular Mechanisms of Age-Related Hearing Loss." *Ageing Research Reviews* 1 (2002): 331–343.

INFORMATION ON SLEEP AND THE BRAIN

Chee, M.W.L., and W. C. Choo. "Functional Imaging of Working Memory After 24 Hr of Total Sleep Deprivation." *Journal of Neuroscience* 24 (2004): 4560–4567.

Gottselig, J. M., G. Hofer-Tinguely, A. A. Borbely, S. J. Regel, H. P. Landolt, J. V. Retey, and P. Achermann. "Sleep and Rest Facilitate Auditory Learning." *Neuroscience* 127 (2004): 557–561.

Guzman-Marin, R., N. Suntsova, M. Methippara, R. Greiffenstein, R. Szymusiak, and D. McGinty. "Sleep Deprivation Suppresses Neurogenesis in the Adult Hippocampus of Rats." *European Journal of Neuroscience* 22 (2005): 2111–2116.

Kavanau, J. L. "Memory, Sleep and the Mechanisms of Synaptic Efficacy Maintenance." *Neuroscience* 79 (1997): 7–44.

Kavanau, J. L. "REM and NREM Sleep as Natural Accompaniments of the Evolution of Warm-Bloodedness." *Neuroscience and Biobehavioral Reviews* 26 (2002): 889–906.

Kavanau, J. L. "Vertebrates That Never Sleep: Implications for Sleep's Basic Function." *Brain Research Bulletin* 46 (1998): 269–279.

Miyamoto, H., and T. K. Hensch. "Reciprocal Interaction of Sleep and Synaptic Plasticity." *Molecular Intervention* 3 (2003): 404–417

INFORMATION ON INSULIN METABOLISM AND BRAIN FUNCTION

Biessels, G. J., B. Bravenboer, and W. H. Gispen. "Glucose, Insulin and the Brain: Modulation of Cognition and Synaptic Plasticity in Health and Disease: A Preface." *European Journal of Pharmacology* 490 (2004): 1–4.

Buren, J., and J. W. Eriksson. "Is Insulin Resistance Caused by Defects in Insulin's Target Cells or by a Stressed Mind?" *Diabetes/Metabolism Research and Reviews* 21 (2005): 487–494.

Carro, E., and I. Torres-Aleman. "The Role of Insulin and Insulin-like Growth Factor 1 in the Molecular and Cellular Mechanisms Underlying the Pathology of Alzheimer's Disease." *European Journal of Pharmacology* 490 (2004):127–133.

Convit, A. "Links Between Cognitive Impairment in Insulin Resistance: An Explanatory Model." *Neurobiology of Aging* 26S (2005): S31–S35.

Convit, A., O. T. Wolf, C. Tarshish, and M. J. de Leon. "Reduced Glucose Tolerance Is Associated with Poor Memory Performance and Hippocampal

Atrophy Among Normal Elderly." *Proceedings of the National Academy of Sciences of the United States of America* 100 (2003): 2019–2022.

Craft, S. "Insulin Resistance and Cognitive Impairment." *Archives of Neurology* 62 (2005): 1043–1044.

Craft, S. "Insulin Resistance Syndrome and Alzheimer's Disease: Age- and Obesity-Related Effects on Memory, Amyloid and Inflammation." *Neurobiology of Aging* 26S (2005): S65–S69.

Craft, S., and G. S. Watson. "Insulin and Neurodegenerative Disease: Shared and Specific Mechanisms." *Lancet* 3 (2004): 169–178.

Fishel, M. A., G. S. Watson, T. J. Montine, Q. Wang, P. S. Green, J. J. Kulstad, D. G. Cook, E. R. Peskind, L. D. Baker, D. Goldgaber, W. Nie, S. Asthana, S. R. Plymate, S. W. Schwartz, and S. Craft. "Hyperinsulinemia Provokes Synchronous Increases in Central Inflammation and β-Amyloid in Normal Adults." *Archives of Neurology* 62 (2005): 1539–1544.

Freude, S., L. Plum, J. Schnitker, U. Leeser, M. Udelhoven, W. Krone, J. C. Bruning, and M. Schubert. "Peripheral Hyperinsulinemia Promotes Tau Phosphorylation in Vivo." *Diabetes* 54 (2005): 3343–3348.

Gasparini, L., W. J. Netzer, P. Greengard, and H. Xu. "Does Insulin Dysfunction Play a Role in Alzheimer's Disease?" *Trends in Pharmacological Sciences* 23 (2002): 288–293.

Gasparini, L., and H. Xu. "Potential Roles of Insulin and IGF-1 in Alzheimer's Disease." *Trends in Neurosciences* 26 (2003): 404–406.

Geroldi, C., G. B. Frisoni, G. Paolisso, S. Bandinelli, J. M. Guralnik, and L. Ferrucci. "Insulin Resistance in Cognitive Impairment." *Archives of Neurology* 62 (2005): 1067–1072.

Gribble, F. M. "A Higher Power for Insulin." *Nature* 434 (2005): 965–966.

Hashizume, K., S. Suzuki, M. Hara, A. Komatsu, and K. Yamashita. "Metabolic Syndrome and Age-Related Dementia: Endocrinological Aspects of Adaptation to Aging." *Mechanisms of Ageing and Development* 127 (2006): 507–510.

Henderson, S. T. "High Carbohydrate Diets and Alzheimer's Disease." *Medical Hypotheses* 62 (2004): 689–700.

Ho, L., W. Qin, P. N. Pompl, Z. Xiang, J. Wang, Z. Zhao, Y. Peng, G. Cambareri, A. Rocher, C. V. Mobbs, P. R. Hof, and G. M. Pasinetti. "Diet-Induced Insulin Resistance Promotes Amyloidosis in a Transgenic Mouse Model of Alzheimer's Disease." *FASEB Journal* 18 (2004): 902–904.

Hong, M., and V.M.Y. Lee. "Insulin and Insulin-like Growth Factor-1 Regulate Tau Phosphorylation in Cultured Human Neurons." *Journal of Biological Chemistry* 272 (1997): 19547–19533.

Lester-Coll, N., E. J. Rivera, S. J. Soscia, K. Doiron, J. R. Wands, and S. M. de la Monte. "Intracerebral Streptozotocin Model of Type 3 Diabetes: Relevance to Sporadic Alzheimer's Disease." *Journal of Alzheimer's Disease* 9 (2006): 13–33.

Luchsinger, J. A., M. X. Tang, S. Shea, and R. Mayeux. "Hyperinsulinemia and Risk of Alzheimer Disease." *Neurology* 63 (2004): 1187–1192.

Martos, R., M. Valle, R. Morales, R. Canete, M. I. Gavilan, and V. Sanchez-Margalet. "Hyperhomocysteinemia Correlates with Insulin Resistance and Low-Grade Systemic Inflammation in Obese Prepubertal Children." *Metabolism* 55 (2006): 72–77.

McCall, A. L. "Altered Glycemia and Brain-Update and Potential Relevance to the Aging Brain." *Neurobiology of Aging* 26S (2005): S70–S75.

Nelson, T. J, and D. L. Alkon. "Insulin and Cholesterol Pathways in Neuronal Function, Memory and Neurodegeneration." *Biochemistry Society Transactions* 33 (2005): 1033–1036.

Rasgon, N. L., and H. A. Kenna. "Insulin Resistance in Depressive Disorders and Alzheimer's Disease: Revisiting the Missing Link Hypothesis." *Neurobiology of Aging* 26S (2005): S103–S107.

Reger, M. A., G. S. Watson, W. H. Frey, L. D. Baker, B. Cholerton, M. L. Keeling, D. A. Belongia, M. A. Fishel, S. R. Plymate, G. D. Schellenberg, M. M. Cherrier, and S. Craft. "Effects of Intranasal Insulin on Cognition in Memory-Impaired Older Adults: Modulation by APOE Genotype." *Neurobiology of Aging* 27 (2006): 451–458.

Risner, M. E., A. M. Saunders, J.F.B. Altman, G. C. Ormandy, S. Craft, I. M. Foley, M. E. Zvartu-Hind, D. A. Hosford, and A. D. Roses. "Efficacy of Rosiglitazone in a Genetically Defined Population with Mild-to-Moderate Alzheimer's Disease." *Pharmacogenomics Journal* 6 (2006): 222–224.

Salkovic-Petrisic, M., F. Tribl, M. Schmidt, S. Hoyer, and P. Riederer. "Alzheimer-like Changes in Protein Kinase B and Glycogen Synthase Kinase-3 in Rat Frontal Cortex and Hippocampus After Damage to the Insulin Signaling Pathway." *Journal of Neurochemistry* 96 (2006): 1005–1015.

Schubert, M., D. Gautam, D. Surjo, K. Ueki, S. Baudler, D. Schubert, T. Kono, J. Abler, N. Galldiks, E. Ulsterman, S. Arndt, A. H. Jacobs, W. Crone, C. R.

Kahn, and J. C. Bruning. "Role for Neuronal Insulin Resistance in Neuro-degenerative Diseases." *Proceedings of the National Academy of Sciences of the United States of America* 101 (2004): 3100–3105.

Steen, E., B. M. Terry, E. J. Rivera, J. L. Cannon, T. R. Neely, R. Tavares, X. J. Xu, J. R. Wands, and S. M. de la Monte. "Impaired Insulin and Insulin-like Growth Factor Expression and Signaling Mechanisms in Alzheimer's Disease—Is This Type 3 Diabetes?" *Journal of Alzheimer's Disease* 7 (2005): 63–80.

Strachan, M.W.J. "Insulin and Cognitive Function in Humans: Experimental Data and Therapeutic Considerations." *Biochemistry Society Transactions* 33 (2005): 1037–1040.

Wada, A., H. Yokoo, T. Yanagita, and H. Kobayashi. "New Twist on Neuronal Insulin Receptor Signaling in Health, Disease and Therapeutics." *Journal of Pharmacological Sciences* 99 (2005): 128–143.

Watson, G. S., and S. Craft. "Insulin Resistance, Inflammation and Cognition in Alzheimer's Disease: Lessons for Multiple Sclerosis." *Journal of Neurological Sciences* 245 (2006): 21–33.

Watson, G. S., and S. Craft. "Modulation of Memory by Insulin and Glucose: Neuropsychological Observations in Alzheimer's Disease." *European Journal of Pharmacology* 490 (2004): 97–113.

Yaffe, K., A. Kanaya, K. Lindquist, E. M. Simonsick, T. Harris, R. I. Shorr, F. A. Tylavsky, and A. B. Newman. "The Metabolic Syndrome, Inflammation and Risk of Cognitive Decline." *Journal of the American Medical Association* 292 (2004): 2237–2242.

INFORMATION ON HIBERNATION, HYPOTHERMIA, AND STARVATION

Avila, J., and J. Diaz-Nido. "Tangling with Hypothermia." *Nature Medicine* 10 (2004): 460–461.

Arendt, T., J. Stieler, A. M. Strijkstra, R. A. Hut, J. Rudiger, E. A. Van der Zee, T. Harkany, M. Holzer, and W. Hartig. "Reversible Paired Helical Filament-like Phosphorylation of Tau Is an Adaptive Process Associated with Neuronal Plasticity in Hibernating Animals." *Journal of Neurosciences* 23 (2003): 6972–6981.

Yanagisawa, M., E. Planel, K. Ishiguro, and S. C. Fujita. "Starvation Induces Tau Phosphorylation in Mouse Brain: Implications for Alzheimer's Disease." *FEBS Letters* 461 (1999): 329–333.

INFORMATION ON KETONE BODIES, KETOGENESIS, AND MEDIUM-CHAIN TRIGLYCERIDES

Cullingford, T. E. "The Ketogenic Diet: Fatty Acids, Fatty Acid-Activated Receptors and Neurological Disorders." *Prostaglandins, Leukotrienes and Essential Fatty Acids* 70 (2004): 253–264

Cunnane, S. C. "Metabolic and Health Implications of Moderate Ketosis and the Ketogenic Diet." *Prostaglandins, Leukotrienes and Essential Fatty Acids* 70 (2004): 233–234.

Cunnane, S. C. "Metabolism of Polyunsaturated Fatty Acids and Ketogenesis: An Emerging Connection." *Prostaglandins, Leukotrienes and Essential Fatty Acids* 70 (2004): 237–241.

Daikhin, Y., and M. Yudkoff. "Ketone Bodies and Brain Glutamate and GABA Metabolism." *Developmental Neuroscience* 20 (1998): 358–364.

Freemantle, E., M. Vandal, J. Tremblay-Mercier, S. Tremblay, J. C. Blachere, M. E. Begin, J. T. Brenna, A. Windust, and S. C. Cunnane. "Omega-3 Fatty Acids, Energy Substrates and Brain Function During Aging." *Prostaglandins, Leukotrienes and Essential Fatty Acids* 75 (2006): 213–220.

Haas, R. H., M. A. Rice, D. A. Trauner, and T. A. Merritt. "Therapeutic Effects of a Ketogenic Diet in Rett Syndrome." *American Journal of Medical Genetics, Supplement* 1 (1986): 225–246.

Massieu, L., M. L. Haces, T. Montiel, and K. Hernandez-Fonseca. "Acetoacetate Protects Hippocampal Neurons Against Glutamate-Mediated Neuronal Damage During Glycolysis Inhibition." *Neuroscience* 120 (2003): 365–378.

Murphy, R., S. Likhodii, K. Nylen, and W. M. Burnham. "The Antidepressant Properties of the Ketogenic Diet." *Biological Psychiatry* 56 (2004): 981–983.

Nebeling, L. C., and E. Lerner. "Implementing a Ketogenic Diet Based on Medium-Chain Triglyceride Oil in Pediatric Patients with Cancer." *Journal of the American Dietetic Association* 95 (1995): 693–697.

Plum, L., M. Schubert, and J. C. Bruning. "The Role of Insulin Receptor Signaling in the Brain." *Trends in Endocrinology and Metabolism* 16 (2005): 59–65.

Reger, M. A., S. T. Henderson, C. Hale, B. Cholerton, L. D. Baker, G. S. Watson, K. Hyde, D. Chapman, and S. Craft. "Effects of Beta-Hydroxybutyrate on Cognition in Memory-Impaired Adults." *Neurobiology of Aging* 25 (2004): 311–314.

Van der Auwera, I., S. Wera, F. Van Leuven, and S. T. Henderson. "A Ketogenic

Diet Reduces Amyloid Beta 40 and 42 in a Mouse Model of Alzheimer's Disease." *Nutrition & Metabolism [London]* 2 (2005): 28.

Veech, R. L. "The Therapeutic Implications of Ketone Bodies: The Effects of Ketone Bodies in Pathological Conditions: Ketogenic Diet, Redox States, Insulin Resistance and Mitochondrial Metabolism." *Prostaglandins, Leukotrienes and Essential Fatty Acids* 70 (2004): 309–319.

Veech, R. L., B. Chance, Y. Kashiwaya, H. A. Lardy, and G. F. Cahill Jr. "Ketone Bodies, Potential Therapeutic Uses." *IUBMB Life* 51 (2001): 241–247.

Yudkoff, M., Y. Daikhin, I. Nissim, O. Horyn, A. Lazarow, B. Luhovyy, S. Wehrli, and I. Nissim. "Response of Brain Amino Acid Metabolism to Ketosis." *Neurochemistry International* 47 (2005): 119–128.

INFORMATION ON DRUG USE AND THE BRAIN

Iacovelli, L., F. Fulceri, A. De Blasi, F. Nicoletti, S. Ruggieri, and F. Fornai. "The Neurotoxicity of Amphetamines: Bridging Drugs of Abuse and Neurodegenerative Disorders." *Experimental Neurology* 201 (2006): 24–31.

Messinis, L., A. Kyprianidou, S. Malefaki, and P. Papathanasopoulos. "Neuropsychological Deficits in Long-Term Frequent Cannabis Users." *Neurology* 66 (2006): 737–739.

Parrott, A. C., and J. Lasky. "Ecstasy (MDMA) Effects Upon Mood and Cognition Before, During and After a Saturday Night Dance." *Psychopharmacology [Berlin]* 139 (1998): 261–268.

Parrott, A. C., A. Lees, N. J. Garnham, M. Jones, and K. Wesnes. "Cognitive Performance in Recreational Users of MDMA (Ecstasy): Evidence for Memory Deficits." *Journal of Psychopharmacology* 12 (1998): 79–83.

Zakzanis, K. K., and Z. Campbell. "Memory Impairment in Now Abstinent MDMA Users and Continued Users: A Longitudinal Follow-up." *Neurology* 66 (2006): 740–741.

INFORMATION ON POLLUTION, SMOKING, AND BRAIN HEALTH

Calderon-Garciduenas, L., W. Reed, R. R. Maronpot, C. Henriquez-Roldan, R. Delgado-Chavez, A. Calderon-Garciduenas, I. Dragustinovis, M. Franco-Lira, M. Aragon-Flores, A. C. Solt, M. Altenberg, R. Torres-Jardon, and J. A. Swenberg. "Brain Inflammation and Alzheimer's-like Pathology in Individuals Exposed to Sever Air Pollution." *Toxicologic Pathology* 32 (2004): 650–658.

Fried, P. A., B. Watkinson, and R. Gray. "Neurocognitive Consequences of

Cigarette Smoking in Young Adults: A Comparison with Pre-Drug Performance." *Neurotoxicology Teratology* 28 (2006): 517–525.

Hill, R. D., L. G. Nilsson, L. Nyberg, and L. Backman. "Cigarette Smoking and Cognitive Performance in Healthy Swedish Adults." *Age and Ageing* 32 (2003): 548–550.

Jacobsen, L. K., J. H. Krystal, W. E. Mencl, M. Westerveld, S. J. Frost, and K. R. Pugh. "Effects of Smoking and Smoking Abstinence on Cognition in Adolescent Tobacco Smokers." *Biological Psychiatry* 57 (2005): 56–66.

Ott, A., K. Andersen, M. E. Dewey, L. Letenneur, C. Brayne, J.R.M. Copeland, J. F. Dartigues, P. Kragh-Sorensen, A. Lobo, J. M. Martinez-Lage, T. Stijnen, A. Hofman, and L. J. Launer. "Effect of Smoking on Global Cognitive Function in Nondemented Elderly." *Neurology* 62 (2004): 920–924.

Paul, R. H., A. M. Brickman, R. A. Cohen, L. M. Williams, R. Niaura, S. Pogun, C. R. Clark, J. Gunstad, and E. Gordon. "Cognitive Status of Young and Older Cigarette Smokers: Data from the International Brain Database." *Journal of Clinical Neuroscience* 13 (2006): 457–465.

Richards, M., M. J. Jarvis, N. Thompson, and M.E.J. Wadsworth. "Cigarette Smoking and Cognitive Decline in Midlife: Evidence from a Prospective Birth Cohort Study." *American Journal of Public Health* 93 (2003): 994–998.

INFORMATION ON EXERCISE, ACTIVITY, AND THE BRAIN

Adlard, P. A., V. M. Perreau, V. Pop, and C. W. Cotman. "Voluntary Exercise Decreases Amyloid Load in a Transgenic Model of Alzheimer's Disease." *Journal of Neuroscience* 25 (2005): 4217–4221.

Barbour, K. A., and J. A. Blumenthal. "Exercise Training and Depression in Older Adults." *Neurobiology of Aging* 26S (2005): S119–S123.

Cobain, M. R., and J. P. Foreyt. "Designing 'Lifestyle Interventions' with the Brain in Mind." *Neurobiology of Aging* 26, suppl. 1 (2005): 85–87.

Gomez-Pinilla, F., Z. Ying, R. R. Roy, R. Molteni, and V. R. Edgerton. "Voluntary Exercise Induces a BDNF-Mediated Mechanism That Promotes Neuroplasticity." *Journal of Neurophysiology* 88 (2002): 2187–2195.

Kramer, A. F., S. J. Colcombe, E. McAuley, P. E. Scalf, and K. I. Erickson. "Fitness, Aging and Neurocognitive Function." *Neurobiology of Aging* 26S (2005): S124–S127.

Lawlor, D. A., and S. W. Hopker. "The Effectiveness of Exercise as an Intervention in the Management of Depression: Systematic Review and Meta-Regression Analysis of Randomized Controlled Trials." *British Medical Journal* 322 (2001): 1–8.

Mattson, M. P., S. L. Chan, and W. Duan. "Modification of Brain Aging and Neurodegenerative Disorders by Genes, Diet and Behavior." *Physiological Reviews* 82 (2002): 637–672.

Parnpiansil, P., N. Jutapakdeegul, T. Chentanez, and N. Kotchabhakdi. "Exercise During Pregnancy Increases Hippocampal Brain-Derived Neurotrophic mRNA Expression and Spatial Learning in Neonatal Rat Pup." *Neuroscience Letters* 352 (2003): 45–48.

Rovio, S., I. Kareholt, E. L. Helkala, M. Viitanen, B. Winblad, J. Tuomilehto, H. Soininen, and A. Nissinen. "Leisure-Time Physical Activity at Midlife and the Risk of Dementia and Alzheimer's Disease." *Lancet Neurology* 4 (2005): 705–711.

Wang, L., E. B. Larson, J. D. Bowen, and G. van Belle. "Performance-based Physical Function and Future Dementia in Older People." *Archives of Internal Medicine* 166 (2006): 1115–1120.

Watson, G. S., M. A. Reger, L. D. Baker, M. J. McNeely, W. Y. Fujimoto, S. E. Kahn, E. J. Boyko, D. L. Leonetti, and S. Craft. "Effects of Exercise and Nutrition on Memory in Japanese Americans with Impaired Glucose Tolerance." *Diabetes Care* 29 (2006): 135–136.

INFORMATION ON COGNITIVE ACTIVITY AND BRAIN HEALTH

Ball, K., D. B. Berch, K. F. Helmers, J. B. Jobe, M. D. Leveck, M. Marsiske, J. N. Morris, G. W. Rebok, D. M. Smith, S. L. Tennstedt, F. W. Unverzagt, and S. L. Willis. "Effects of Cognitive Training Interventions with Older Adults." *Journal of the American Medical Association* 288 (2002): 2271–2281.

Borzekowski, D.L.G., and T. N. Robinson. "The Remote, the Mouse, and the Number 2 Pencil: The Household Media Environment and Academic Achievement Among Third Grade Students." *Archives of Pediatrics & Adolescent Medicine* 159 (2005): 607–613.

Erickson, K. I., S. J. Colcombe, R. Wadhwa, L. Bherer, M. S. Peterson, P. E. Scalf, J. S. Kim, M. Alvarado, and A. F. Kramer. "Training-Induced Plasticity in Older Adults: Effects of Training on Hemispheric Asymmetry." *Neurobiology of Aging* (forthcoming).

Fritsch, T., K. A. Smyth, S. M. Dubanne, G. J. Petot, and R. P. Friedland. "Participation in Novelty-Seeking Leisure Activities and Alzheimer's Disease." *Journal of Geriatric Psychiatry and Neurology* 18 (2005): 134–141.

Hancox, R. J., B. J. Milne, and R. Poulton. "Association of Television Viewing During Childhood with Poor Educational Achievement." *Archives of Pediatrics & Adolescent Medicine* 159 (2005): 614–618.

Hultsch, D., C. Hertzog, B. Small, and R. Dixon. "Use It or Lose It: Engaged Lifestyle as a Buffer of Cognitive Decline in Aging?" *Psychology of Aging* 14 (1999): 245–263.

Kondo, Y., M. Suzuki, S. Mugikura, N. Abe, S. Takahashi, T. Iijima, and T. Fujii. "Changes in Brain Activation Associated with Use of a Memory Strategy: A Functional MRI Study." *NeuroImage* 24 (2005): 1154–1163.

May, A., G. Hajak, S. Gransbauer, T. Steffens, B. Langguth, T. Kleinjung, and P. Eichhammer. "Structural Brain Alterations Following 5 Days of Intervention: Dynamic Aspects of Neuroplasticity." *Cerebral Cortex* (forthcoming).

Nyberg, L., J. Sandblom, S. Jones, A. S. Neely, K. M. Petersson, M. Ingvar, and L. Backman. "Neural Correlates of Training-Related Memory Improvement in Adulthood and Aging." *Proceedings of the National Academy of Sciences of the United States of America* 100 (2003): 13728–13733.

Rundek, T., and D. A. Bennett. "Cognitive Leisure Activities, But Not Watching TV, for Future Brain Benefits." *Neurology* 66 (2006): 794–795.

Wilson, R. S., D. A. Bennett, D. W. Gilley, L. A. Beckett, L. L. Barnes, and D. A. Evans. "Premorbid Reading Activity and Patterns of Cognitive Decline in Alzheimer Disease." *Archives of Neurology* 57 (2000): 1718–1723.

Wilson, R. S., C.F.M. de Leon, L. L. Barnes, J. A. Schneider, J. L. Bienias, D. A. Evans, and D. A. Bennett. "Participation in Cognitively Stimulating Activities and Risk of Incident Alzheimer Disease." *Journal of the American Medical Association* 287 (2002): 742–748.

Zimmerman, F. J., and D. A. Christakis. "Children's Television Viewing and Cognitive Outcomes." *Archives Pediatrics & Adolescent Medicine* 159 (2005): 619–625.

INFORMATION ON NEUROIMAGING

Bellec, P., V. Perlbarg, S. Jbabdi, M. Pelegrini-Isaac, J. L. Anton, J. Doyon, and H. Benali. "Identification of Large-Scale Networks in the Brain Using fMRI." *NeuroImage* 29 (2006): 1231–1243.

Blasi, G., T. E. Goldberg, T. Weickert, S. Das, P. Kohn, B. Zoltick, A. Bertolino, J. H. Callicott, D. R. Weinberger, and V. S. Mattay. "Brain Regions Underlying Inhibition and Interference Monitoring and Suppression." *European Journal of Neuroscience* 23 (2006): 1658–1664.

Bookheimer, S. Y., M. H. Strojwas, M. S. Cohen, A. M. Saunders, M. A. Pericak-Vance, J. C. Mazziotta, and G. W. Small. "Patterns of Brain Activation in People at Risk for Alzheimer's Disease." *New England Journal of Medicine* 343 (2000): 450–456.

Buckner, R. L., A. Z. Snyder, B. J. Shannon, G. LaRossa, R. Sachs, A. F. Fotenos, Y. I. Sheline, W. E. Klunk, C. A. Mathis, J. C. Morris, and M. A. Mintun. "Molecular, Structural and Functional Characterization of Alzheimer's Disease: Evidence for a Relationship Between Default Activity, Amyloid and Memory." *Journal of Neuroscience* 25 (2005): 7709–7717.

Cavanna, A. E., and M. R. Trimble. "The Precuneus: A Review of its Functional Anatomy and Behavioral Correlates." *Brain* 129 (2006): 564–583.

Chao, L. L., and R. T. Knight. "Prefrontal Deficits in Attention and Inhibitory Control with Aging." *Cerebral Cortex* 7 (1997): 63–69.

Den Heijer, T., P. E. Sijens, N. D. Prins, A. Hofman, P. J. Koudstaal, M. Oudkerk, and M.M.B. Breteler. "MR Spectroscopy of the Brain White Matter in the Prediction of Dementia." *Neurology* 66 (2006): 540–544.

Fox, M. D., A. Z. Snyder, J. L. Vincent, M. Corbetta, D. C. Van Essen, and M. E. Raichle. "The Human Brain Is Intrinsically Organized into Dynamic, Anti-correlated Functional Networks." *Proceedings of the National Academy of Sciences of the United States of America* 102 (2005): 9673–9678.

Gazzaley, A., and M. D'Esposito. "The Contribution of Functional Brain Imaging to Our Understanding of Cognitive Aging." *Science of Aging Knowledge Environment* 4 (2003): PE2.

Greicius, M. D., B. Krasnow, A. L. Reiss, and V. Menon. "Functional Connectivity in the Resting Brain: A Network Analysis of the Default Mode Hypothesis." *Proceedings of the National Academy of Sciences of the United States of America* 100 (2003): 253–258.

Greicius, M. D., G. Srivastava, A. L. Reiss, and V. Menon. "Default-Mode Activity Distinguishes Alzheimer's Disease from Healthy Aging: Evidence from Functional MRI." *Proceedings of the National Academy of Sciences of the United States of America* 101 (2004): 4637–4642.

Gusnard, D. A., E. Akbudak, G. L. Shulman, and M. E. Raichle. "Medial Prefrontal

Cortex and Self-Referential Mental Activity: Relation to a Default Mode of Brain Function." *Proceedings of the National Academy of Sciences of the United States of America* 98 (2001): 4259–4264.

Johnson, S. C., T. W. Schmitz, C. H. Moritz, C. H. Meyerand, H. A. Rowley, A. L. Alexander, K. W. Hanen, C. E. Gleason, C. M. Carlsson, M. L. Ries, S. Asthana, K. Chen, E. M. Reiman, and G. E. Alexander. "Activation of Brain Regions Vulnerable to Alzheimer's Disease: The Effect of Mild Cognitive Impairment." *Neurobiology of Aging* 27 (2006): 1604–1612.

Lind, J., A. Larsson, J. Persson, M. Ingvar, L. G. Nilsson, L. Backman, R. Adolfsson, M. Cruts, K. Sleegers, C. Van Broeckhoven, and L. Nyberg. "Reduced Hippocampal Volume in Non-Demented Carriers of the Apolipoprotein E Epsilon 4: Relation to Chronological Age and Recognition Memory." *Neuroscience Letters* 396 (2006): 23–27.

Lustig, C., A. Z. Snyder, M. Bhakta, K. C. O'Brien, M. McAvoy, M. E. Raichle, J. C. Morris, and R. L. Buckner. "Functional Deactivations: Change with Age and Dementia of the Alzheimer Type." *Proceedings of the National Academy of Sciences of the United States of America* 100 (2003): 14504–14509.

McNally, R. J. "Cognitive Abnormalities in Post-Traumatic Stress Disorder." *Trends in Cognitive Science* 10 (2006): 271–277.

O'Sullivan, M., D. K. Jones, P. E. Summers, R. G. Morris, S.C.R. Williams, and H. S. Markus. "Evidence for Cortical 'Disconnection' as a Mechanism of Age-Related Cognitive Decline." *Neurology* 57 (2001): 632–638.

Pliszka, S. R., D. C. Glahn, M. Semrud-Clikeman, C. Franklin, R. Perez III, J. Xiong, and M. Liotti. "Neuroimaging of Inhibitory Control Areas in Children with Attention Deficit Hyperactivity Disorder Who Were Treatment Naïve or in Long-Term Treatment." *American Journal of Psychiatry* 163 (2006): 1052–1060.

Raichle, M. E. "Functional Brain Imaging and Human Brain Function." *Journal of Neurosciences* 23 (2003): 3959–3962.

Raichle, M. E., A. M. MacLeod, A. Z. Snyder, W. J. Powers, D. A. Gusnard, and G. L. Shulman. "A Default Mode of Brain Function." *Proceedings of the National Academy of Sciences of the United States of America* 98 (2001): 676–682.

Reiman, E. M., K. Chen, G. E. Alexander, R. J. Caselli, D. Bandy, D. Osborne, A. Saunders, and J. Hardy. "Functional Brain Abnormalities in Young Adults at Genetic Risk for Late-Onset Alzheimer's Dementia." *Proceedings of the National Academy of Sciences of the United States of America* 101 (2004): 284–289.

Sharp, D. J., S. K. Scott, M. A. Mehta, and R.J.S. Wise. "The Neural Correlates of Declining Performance with Age: Evidence for Age-Related Changes in Cognitive Control." *Cerebral Cortex* (forthcoming).

Smith, A. B., E. Taylor, M. Brammer, B. Toone, and K. Rubia. "Task-Specific Hypoactivation in Prefrontal and Temporoparietal Brain Regions During Motor Inhibition and Task Switching in Medication-Naive Children and Adolescents with Attention Deficit Hyperactivity Disorder." *American Journal of Psychiatry* 163 (2006): 1044–1051.

Springer, M. V., A. R. McIntosh, G. Winocur, and C. L. Grady. "The Relation Between Brain Activity During Memory Tasks and Years of Education in Young and Older Adults." *Neuropsychology* 19 (2005): 181–192.

Tamm, L., V. Menon, and A. L. Reiss. "Parietal Attentional System Aberrations During Target Detection in Adolescents with Attention Deficit Hyperactivity Disorder: Event-Related fMRI Evidence." *American Journal of Psychiatry* 163 (2006): 1033–1043.

Van den Heuvel, D.M.J., V. H. ten Dam, A.J.M. de Craen, F. Admiraal-Behloul, H. Olofsen, E.L.E.M. Bollen, J. Jolles, H. M. Murray, G. J. Blauw, R.G.J. Westendorp, and M. A. van Buchem. "Increase in Periventricular White Matter Hyperintensities Parallels Decline in Mental Processing Speed in a Non-Demented Elderly Population." *Journal of Neurology, Neurosurgery, and Psychiatry* 77 (2006): 149–153.

INFORMATION ON HOT FLASHES AND HORMONES

Bagger, Y. Z., L. B. Tanko, P. Alexandersen, G. Qin, and C. Christiansen. "Early Postmenopausal Hormone Therapy May Prevent Cognitive Impairment Later in Life." *Menopause* 12 (2005): 12–17.

Bishop, J., and J. W. Simpkins. "Estradiol Enhances Brain Glucose Uptake in Ovariectomized Rats." *Brain Research Bulletin* 36 (1995): 315–320.

Borg, W. P., M. J. During, R. S. Sherwin, M. A. Borg, M. L. Brines, and G. L. Shulman. "Ventromedial Hypothalamic Lesions in Rats Suppress Counter-regulatory Responses to Hypoglycemia." *Journal of Clinical Investigation* 93 (1994): 1677–1682.

Dormire, S. L., and N. K. Reame. "Menopausal Hot Flash Frequency Changes in Response to Experimental Manipulation of Blood Glucose." *Nursing Research* 52 (2003): 338–343.

El-Tayeb, K. M., P. L. Brubaker, H. L. Lickley, E. Cook, and M. Vranic. "Effect of

Opiate-Receptor Blockade on Normoglycemic and Hypoglycemic Glucoregulation." *American Journal of Physiology* 250 (1986): E236–E242.

Fitzpatrick, L. A., and R. J. Santen. "Hot Flashes: The Old and the New, What Is Really True." *Mayo Clinic Proceedings* 77 (2002): 1155–1158.

Freedman, R. R. "Biochemical, Metabolic and Vascular Mechanisms in Menopausal Hot Flashes." *Fertility and Sterility* 70 (1998): 332–337.

Freedman, R. R. "Pathophysiology and Treatment of Menopausal Hot Flashes." *Seminars in Reproductive Medicine* 23 (2005): 117–125.

Gennazzani, A. R., M. Stomata, F. Bernardi, S. Luisi, E. Casarosa, S. Puccetti, A. D. Gennazzani, M. Palumbo, and M. Luisi. "Conjugated Equine Estrogens Reverse the Effects of Aging on Central and Peripheral Allopregnanolone and Beta-Endorphin Levels in Female Rats." *Fertility and Sterility* 81, suppl. 1 (2004): 757–766.

Guthrie, J. R., L. Dennerstein, J. R. Taffe, P. Lehert, and H. G. Burger. "Hot Flushes During the Menopause Transition: A Longitudinal Study in Australian-Born Women." *Menopause* 12 (2005): 460–467.

Guttuso Jr., T. J. "Gabapentin's Effects on Hot Flashes and Hypothermia." *Neurology* 54 (2000): 2161–2163.

Guttuso Jr., T. J. "Hot Flashes Refractory to HRT and SSRI Therapy but Responsive to Gabapentin Therapy." *Journal of Pain and Symptom Management* 27 (2004): 274–276.

Harmon, S. M., F. Naftolin, E. A. Brinton, and D. R. Judelson. "Is the Estrogen Controversy Over? Deconstructing the Women's Health Initiative Study: A Critical Evaluation of the Evidence." *Annals of the New York Academy of Science* 1052 (2005): 43–56.

Henderson, V. W. "Only a Matter of Time? Hormone Therapy and Cognition." *Menopause* 12 (2005): 1–3.

Jeffrey, S. M., J. J. Pepe, L. M. Popovich, and G. Vitagliano. "Gabapentin for Hot Flashes in Prostate Cancer." *Annals of Pharmacotherapy* 36 (2002): 433–436.

Katovich, M. J., and J. O'Meara. "Effect of Chronic Estrogen on the Skin Temperature Response to Naloxone in Morphine-Dependent Rats." *Canadian Journal of Physiology and Parmacology* 65 (1987): 563–567.

Katovich, M. J., D. L. Pitman, and C. C. Barney. "Mechanisms Mediating the Thermal Response to Morphine Withdrawal in Rats." *Proceedings of the Society for Experimental Biology and Medicine* 193 (1990): 129–135.

Klepper, J., S. Diefenbach, A. Kohlschutter, and T. Voit. "Effects of the Ketogenic

Diet in the Glucose Transporter 1 Deficiency Syndrome." *Prostaglandins, Leukotrienes, and Essential Fatty Acids* 70 (2004): 321–327.

Leventhal, L., S. Cosmi, and D. Deecher. "Effect of Calcium Channel Modulators on Temperature Regulation in Ovariectomized Rats." *Pharmacology of Biochemistry and Behavoir* 80 (2005): 511–520.

Martinez-Raga, J., A. Sabater, B. Perez-Galvez, M. Castellano, and G. Cervera. "Add-On Gabapentin in the Treatment of Opiate Withdrawal." *Progress in Neuro-Psychopharmacology & Biological Psychiatry* 28 (2004): 599–601.

Molina, P. E., and N. N. Abumrad. "Contribution of Excitatory Amino Acids to Hypoglycemic Counter-Regulation." *Brain Research* 899 (2001): 201–208.

Nakamura, T., D. Yoshihara, T. Ohmori, M. Yanai, and Y. Takeshita. "Effects of Diet High in Medium-Chain Triglyceride on Plasma Ketone, Glucose and Insulin Concentrations in Enterectomized and Normal Rats." *Journal of Nutritional Science and Vitaminology* 40 (1994): 147–159.

Nelson, H. D., K. K. Vesco, E. Haney, R. Fu, A. Nedrow, J. Miller, C. Nicolaidis, M. Walker, and L. Humphrey. "Nonhormonal Therapies for Menopausal Hot Flashes." *Journal of the American Medical Association* 295 (2006): 2057–2071.

Pandya, K. J., G. R. Morrow, J. A. Roscoe, H. Zhao, J. T. Hickok, E. Pajon, T. J. Sweeney, T. K. Banerjee, and P. J. Flynn. "Gabapentin for Hot Flashes in 420 Women with Breast Cancer: A Randomized Double-Blind Placebo-Controlled Trial." *Lancet* 366 (2005): 818–824.

Plecko, B., S. Stoeckler-Ipsiroglu, E. Schober, G. Harrer, V. Mlynarik, S. Gruber, E. Moser, D. Moeslinger, H. Silgoner, and I. Ipsiroglu. "Oral β-Hydroxybutyrate Supplementation in Two Patients with Hyperinsulinemic Hypoglycemia: Monitoring of β-Hydroxybutyrate Levels in Blood and Cerebrospinal Fluid, and in the Brain by *in vivo* Magnetic Resonance Spectroscopy." *Pediatric Research* 52 (2002): 301–306.

Randolph Jr., J. F., M. F. Sowers, I. Bondarenko, E. B. Gold, G. A. Greendale, J. T. Bromberger, S. E. Brockwell, and K. A. Matthews. "The Relationship of Longitudinal Change in Reproductive Hormones and Vasomotor Symptoms During the Menopausal Transition." *Journal of Clinical Endocrinology and Metabolism* 90 (2005): 6106–6112.

Rapkin, A. J. "Vasomotor Symptoms in Menopause: Physiologic Condition and Central Nervous System Approaches to Treatment." *American Journal Obstetrics and Gynecology* (forthcoming).

Rapp, S. R., M. A. Espeland, S. A. Shumaker, V. W. Henderson, R. L. Brunner, J. E. Manson, M.L.S. Gass, M. L. Stefanick, D. S. Lane, J. Hays, K. C. Johnson, L. H. Coker, M. Dailey, and D. Bowen. "Effect of Estrogen Plus Progestin on Global Cognitive Function in Postmenopausal Women. The Women's Health Initiative Memory Study: A Randomized Controlled Trial." *Journal of the American Medical Association* 289 (2003): 2663–2672.

Ratka, A. "Menopausal Hot Flashes and Development of Cognitive Impairment." *Annals of the New York Academy of Science* 1052 (2005): 11–26.

Reddy, S. Y., H. Warner, T. Guttoso Jr., S. Messing, W. DiGrazio, L. Thornberg, and T. S. Guzick. "Gabapentin, Estrogen and Placebo for Treating Hot Flushes." *Obstetrics and Gynecology* 108 (2006): 41–48.

Resnick, S. M., P. M. Maki, S. Golski, M. A. Kraut, and A. B. Zonderman. "Effects of Estrogen Replacement on PET Cerebral Blood Flow and Neuropsychological Performance." *Hormones and Behavior* 34 (1998): 171–182.

Sandoval, D. A., A. C. Ertl, M. A. Richardson, D. B. Tate, and S. N. Davis. "Estrogen Blunts Neuroendocrine and Metabolic Responses to Hypoglycemia." *Diabetes* 52 (2003): 1749–1755.

Segel, S. A., D. S. Paramore, and P. E. Cryer. "Hypoglycemia-Associated Autonomic Failure in Advanced Type 2 Diabetes." *Diabetes* 51 (2002): 724–733.

Shanafelt, T. D., D. L. Barton, A. A. Adjei, and C. L. Loprinzi. "Pathophysiology and Treatment of Hot Flashes." *Mayo Clinic Proceedings* 77 (2002): 1207–1218.

Shi, J., and J. W. Simpkins. "17 β-Estradiol Modulation of Glucose Transporter 1 Expression in Blood-Brain Barrier." *American Journal of Physiology* 272 (1997): E1016–E1022.

Shumaker, S. A., C. Legault, S. R. Rapp, L. Thal, R. B. Wallace, J. K. Ockene, S. L. Hendrix, B. N. Jones III, A. R. Assaf, R. D. Jackson, J. M. Kotchen, S. Wassertheil-Smoller, and J. Wactawski-Wende. "Estrogen Plus Progestin and the Incidence of Dementia and Mild Cognitive Impairment in Postmenopausal Women. The Women's Health Initiative Memory Study: A Randomized Controlled Trial." *Journal of American Medical Association* 289 (2003): 1651–2662.

Simpkins, J. W., D. K. Andreadis, W. J. Millard, and M. J. Katovich. "The Effect of Cellular Glucoprivation on Skin Temperature Regulation in the Rat." *Life Sciences* 47 (1990): 107–115.

Simpkins, J. W., M. J. Katovich, and W. J. Millard. "Glucose Modulation of Skin Temperature Response During Morphine Withdrawal in the Rat." *Psychopharmacology [Berlin]* 102 (1990): 213–220.

Simpkins, J. W., M. J. Katovich, and I. C. Song. "Similarities Between Morphine Withdrawal in the Rat and the Menopausal Hot Flush." *Life Sciences* 32 (1983): 1957–1966.

Stearns, V., L. Ullmer, J. F. Lopez, Y. Smith, C. Isaacs, and D. F. Hayes. "Hot Flushes." *Lancet* 360 (2002): 1851–1861.

Wasserthail-Smoller, S., S. L. Hendrix, M. Limacher, G. Heiss, C. Kooperberg, A. Baird, T. Kotchen, J. D. Curb, H. Black, J. E. Rossouw, A. Aragaki, M. Safford, E. Stein, S. Laowattana, and W. J. Mysiw. "Effect of Estrogen Plus Progestin on Stroke in Postmenopausal Women. The Women's Health Initiative: A Randomized Trial." *Journal of the American Medical Association* 289 (2003): 2673–2684.

Willemsen, M.A.A.P., R. J. Soorani-Lunsing, E. Pouwels, and J. Kleppert. "Neuroglycopenia in Normoglycemic Patients, and the Potential Benefit of Ketosis." *Diabetic Medicine* 20 (2003): 481–482.

Yamada, K. A., N. Rensing, and L. L. Thio. "Ketogenic Diet Reduces Hypoglycemia-Induced Neuronal Death in Young Rats." *Neuroscience Letters* 385 (2005): 210–214.

INFORMATION ON MIGRAINE HEADACHES

Ayata, C., H. Jin, C. Kudo, T. Dalkara, and M. A. Moskowitz. "Suppression of Cortical Spreading Depression in Migraine Prophylaxis." *Annals of Neurology* 59 (2006): 652–661.

Backonja, M. M. "Use of Anticonvulsants for Treatment of Neuropathic Pain." *Neurology* 59 (2002): S14–S17.

Bolay, H., U. Reuter, A. K. Dunn, Z. Huang, D. A. Boas, and M. A. Moskowitz. "Intrinsic Brain Activity Triggers Trigeminal Meningeal Afferents in a Migraine Model." *Nature Medicine* 8 (2002): 136–142.

Bowyer, S. M., S. K. Aurora, J. E. Moran, N. Tepley, and K.M.A. Welch. "Magnetoencephalographic Fields from Patients with Spontaneous and Induced Migraine Aura." *Annals of Neurology* 50 (2001): 582–587.

Buchgreitz, L., A. C. Lyngberg, L. Bendtsen, and R. Jensen. "Frequency of Headache Is Related to Sensitization: A Population Study." *Pain* 123 (2006): 19–27.

Bussone, G. "Pathophysiology of Migraine." *Neurological Sciences* 25 (2004): S239–S241.

D'Andrea, G., G. P. Nordera, and G. Allais. "Treatment of Aura: Solving the Puzzle." *Neurology Sciences* 27 (2006): S96–S99.

Dalkara, T., N. T. Zervas, and M. A. Moskowitz. "From Spreading Depression to the Trigeminovascular System." *Neurological Sciences* 27 (2006): S86–S90.

Del Rio, M. S., and J. A. Linera. "Functional Neuroimaging of Headaches." *Lancet Neurology* 3 (2004): 645–651.

Goadsby, P. J. "Migraine Pathophysiology." *Headache* 45, suppl. 1 (2005): S14–S24.

Hadjikani, N., M. S. del Rio, O. Wu, D. Schwartz, D. Bakker, B. Fischl, K. K. Kwong, F. M. Cutrer, B. R. Rosen, R.B.H. Tootell, A. G. Sorensen, and M. A. Moskowitz. "Mechanisms of Migraine Aura Revealed by Functional MRI in Human Visual Cortex." *Proceedings of the National Academy of Sciences of the United States of America* 98 (2001): 4687–4692.

Iadecola, C. "From CSD to Headache: A Long and Winding Road." *Nature Medicine* 8 (2002): 110–112.

Ji, R. R., T. Kohno, K. A. Moore, and C. J. Woolf. "Central Sensitization and LTP: Do Pain and Memory Share Similar Mechanisms?" *Trends in Neuroscience* 26 (2003): 696–705.

Kato, T. "Role of Magnesium Ions on the Regulation of NMDA Receptor—A Pharmacopathology of Memantine." *Clinical Calcium* 14 (2004): 76–80.

Lipton, R. B., and M. E. Bigal. "Migraine: Epidemiology, Impact and Risk Factors for Progression." *Headache* 45, suppl. 1 (2005): S3–S13.

Loder, E., and D. Biondi. "General Principles of Migraine Management: The Changing Role of Prevention." *Headache* 45, suppl. 1 (2005): S33–S47.

Maneyapanda, S. B., and A. Venkatasubrmanian. "Relationship Between Significant Perinatal Events and Migraine Severity." *Pediatrics* 116 (2005): e555–e558.

Marrannes, R., R. Willems, E. De Prins, and A. Wauquier. "Evidence for a Role of the N-Methyl-D-Aspartate (NMDA) Receptor in Cortical Spreading Depression in the Rat." *Brain Research* 457 (1988): 226–240.

Molnar, P., and S. L. Erdo. "Vinpocetine Is as Potent as Phenytoin to Block Voltage-Gated Na+ Channels in Rat Cortical Neurons." *European Journal of Pharmacology* 273 (1995): 303–306.

Moskowitz, M. A., K. Nozaki, and R. P. Kraig. "Neocortical Spreading Depression Provokes the Expression of *C-fos* Protein-like Immunoreactivity within Trigeminal Nucleus Caudalis Via Trigeminovascular Mechanisms." *Journal of Neurosciences* 13 (1993): 1167–1177.

Mousain-Bosc, M., M. Roche, J. Rapin, and J. P. Bali. "Magnesium Vit B6 Intake Reduces Central Nervous System Hyperexcitability in Children." *Journal of American College of Nutrition* 23 (2004): 545S–548S.

Saugstad, L. F. "A 'New-Old' Way of Thinking About Brain Disorder, Cerebral Excitability—The Fundamental Property of Nervous Tissue." *Medicine Hypotheses* 64 (2005): 142–150.

Schoenen, J. "Neurophysiological Features of the Migrainous Brain." *Neurological Science* 27 (2006): S77–S81.

Strahlman, R. S. "Can Ketosis Help Migraine Sufferers? A Case Report." *Headache* 46 (2006): 182.

Waeber, C., and M. A. Moskowitz. "Therapeutic Implications of Central and Peripheral Mechanisms in Migraine." *Neurology* 61 (2003): S9–S20.

Welch, K. M., and N. M. Ramadan. "Mitochondria, Magnesium and Migraine." *Journal of Neurological Sciences* 134 (1995): 9–14.

Welch, K. M. "Brain Hyperexcitability: The Basis for Antiepileptic Drugs in Migraine Prevention." *Headache* 45, suppl. 1 (2005): S25–S32.

Welch, K. M. "Contemporary Concepts of Migraine Pathogenesis." *Neurology* 61 (2003): S2–S8.

Woods, R. P., M. Iacaboni, and J. C. Mazziotta. "Bilateral Spreading Cerebral Hypoperfusion During Spontaneous Migraine Headache." *New England Journal of Medicine* 331 (1994): 1689–1692.

INFORMATION ON COGNITIVE DECLINE

Aberg, E., C. P. Hofstetter, L. Olson, and S. Brene. "Moderate Ethanol Consumption Increases Hippocampal Cell Proliferation and Neurogenesis in the Adult Mouse." *International Journal of Neuropsychopharmacology* 8 (2005): 557–567.

Ahles, T. A., A. J. Saykin, C. T. Furstenberg, B. Cole, L. A. Mott, K. Skalla, M. B. Whedon, S. Bivens, T. Mitchell, E. R. Greenberg, and P. M. Silberfarb. "Neuropsychologic Impact of Standard-Dose Systemic Chemotherapy in Long-Term Survivors of Breast Cancer and Lymphoma." *Journal of Clinical Oncology* 20 (2002): 485–493.

Algaidi, S. A., L. A. Christie, A. M. Jenkinson, L. Whalley, G. Riedel, and B. Platt.

"Long-term Homocysteine Exposure Induces Alterations in Spatial Learning, Hippocampal Signaling and Synaptic Plasticity." *Experimental Neurology* 197 (2006): 8–21.

Backman, L., N. Ginovart, R. A. Dixon, T.B.R. Wahlin, A. Wahlin, C. Halldin, and L. Farde. "Age-Related Cognitive Deficits Mediated by Changes in the Striatal Dopamine System." *American Journal of Psychiatry* 157 (2000): 635–637.

Bartzokis, G., P. H. Lu, D. H. Geschwind, N. Edwards, J. Mintz, and J. L. Cummings. "Apolioprotein E Genotype and Age-Related Myelin Breakdown in Healthy Individuals: Implications for Cognitive Decline and Dementia." *Archives of General Psychiatry* 63 (2006): 63–72.

Bartzokis, G., T. A. Tishler, P. H. Lu, P. Villablanca, L. L. Altschuler, M. Carter, D. Huang, N. Edwards, and J. Mintz. "Brain Ferritin Iron May Influence Age- and Gender-Related Risks of Neurodegeneration." *Neurobiology of Aging* (forthcoming).

Bodnar, L. M., and K. L. Wisner. "Nutrition and Depression: Implications for Improving Mental Health Among Childbearing-Aged Women." *Biological Psychiatry* 58 (2005): 679–685.

Bronwen, M., M. P. Mattson, and S. Maudsley. "Caloric Restriction and Intermittent Fasting: Two Potential Diets for Successful Brain Aging." *Ageing Research Reviews* 5 (2006): 332–353.

Brookmeyer, B., S. Gray, and C. Kawas. "Projections of Alzheimer's Disease in the United States and the Public Health Impact of Delaying Disease Onset." *American Journal of Public Health* 88 (1998): 1337–1342.

Caselli, R. J., E. M. Reiman, D. Osborne, J. G. Hentz, L. C. Baxter, J. L. Hernandez, and G. G. Alexander. "Longitudinal Changes in Cognition and Behavior in Asymptomatic Carriers of the APO E ε4 Allele." *Neurology* 62 (2004): 1990–1995.

Conde, J. R., and W. J. Streit. "Microglia in the Aging Brain." *Journal of Neuropathology Experimental Neurology* 65 (2006): 19–203.

Cotman, C. W. "The Role of Neurotrophins in Brain Aging: A Perspective in Honor of Regino Perez-Polo." *Neurochemical Research* 30 (2005): 877–881.

Curb, J. D., B. L. Rodriquez, R. D. Abbott, H. Petrovitch, G. W. Ross, K. H. Masaki, D. Foley, P. L. Blanchette, T. Harris, R. Chen, and L. R. White. "Longitudinal Association of Vascular and Alzheimer's Dementias, Diabetes and Glucose Tolerance." *Neurology* 52 (1999): 971–975.

de Magalhaes, J. P., and A. Sandberg. "Cognitive Aging as an Extension of Brain Development: A Model Linking Learning, Brain Plasticity and Neurodegeneration." *Mechanisms of Ageing Development* 126 (2005): 1026–1033.

Den Heijer, T., L. J. Launer, N. D. Prins, E. J. van Dijk, S. E. Vermeer, A. Hofman, P. J. Koudstaal, and M.M.B. Breteler. "Association Between Blood Pressure, White Matter Lesions and Atrophy of the Medial Temporal Lobe." *Neurology* 64 (2005): 263–267.

Devanand, D. P., G. H. Pelton, D. Zamora, X. Liu, M. H. Tabert, M. Goodkind, N. Scarmeas, I. Braun, Y. Stern, and R. Mayeux. "Predictive Utility of Apolipoprotein E Genotype for Alzheimer Disease in Outpatients with Mild Cognitive Impairment." *Archives of Neurology* 62 (2005): 975–980.

Dickerson, B. C., D. H. Salat, D. N. Greve, E. F. Chua, E. Rand-Giovannetti, D. M. Rentz, L. Bertram, K. Mullin, R. E. Tanzi, D. Blacker, M. S. Albert, and R. A. Sperling. "Increased Hippocampal Activation in Mild Cognitive Impairment Compared to Normal Aging and AD." *Neurology* 65 (2005): 404 411.

Ding, Q., S. Vaynman, M. Akhavan, Z. Ying, and F. Gomez-Pinilla. "Insulin-like Growth Factor 1 Interfaces with Brain-Derived Neurotrophic Factor-Mediated Synaptic Plasticity to Modulate Aspects of Exercise-Induced Cognitive Function." *Neuroscience* 140 (2006): 823–833.

Dumas, R. S. "Neurotrophic Factors and Regulation of Mood: Role of Exercise, Diet and Metabolism." *Neurobiology of Aging* 26S (2005): 388–393.

Enzinger, C., F. Fazekas, P. M. Matthews, S. Ropele, H. Schmidt, S. Smith, and R. Schmidt. "Risk Factors for Progression of Brain Atrophy in Aging." *Neurology* 64 (2005): 1704–1711.

Finefrock, A. E., A. I. Bush, and P. M. Doraiswamy. "Current Status of Metals as Therapeutic Targets in Alzheimer's Disease." *Journal of the American Geriatric Society* 51 (2003): 1143–1148.

Fuchs, E., B. Czeh, M.H.P. Kole, T. Michaelis, and P. J. Lucassen. "Alterations in Neuroplasticity in Depression: The Hippocampus and Beyond." *European Neuropsychopharmacology* 14 (2004): S481–S490.

Geda, Y. E., D. S. Knopman, D. A. Mrazek, G. A. Jicha, G. E. Smith, S. Negash, B. F. Boeve, R. J. Ivnik, R. C. Peterson, V. S. Pankratz, and W. A. Rocca. "Depression, Apolipoprotein E Genotype and the Incidence of Mild Cognitive Impairment." *Archives of Neurology* 63 (2006): 435–440.

Green, R. C., L. A. Cupples, A. Kurz, S. Auerbach, R. Go, D. Sadovnick, R. Duara, W. A. Kukull, H. Chui, T. Edeki, P. A. Griffith, R. P. Friedland, D. Bachman, and

L. Farrer. "Depression as a Risk Factor for Alzheimer Disease." *Archives of Neurology* 60 (2003): 753–759.

Hayley, S., M. O. Poulter, Z. Merali, and H. Anisman. "The Pathogenesis of Clinical Depression: Stressor- and Cytokine-Induced Alterations of Neuroplasticity." *Neuroscience* 135 (2005): 659–678.

Heininger, K. "A Unifying Hypothesis of Alzheimer's Disease. III. Risk Factors." *Human Psychopharmacology* 15 (2000): 1–70.

Heininger, K. "A Unifying Hypothesis of Alzheimer's Disease. IV. Causation and Sequence of Events." *Reviews in the Neurosciences* 11 (2000): 213–328.

Helmuth, L. "A Generation Gap in Brain Activity." *Science* 296 (2002): 2131–2133.

Henderson, V. W., K. S. Benke, R. C. Green, L. A. Cupples, and L. A. Farrer for the MIRAGE Study Group. "Postmenopausal Hormone Therapy and Alzheimer's Disease Risk: Interaction with Age." *Journal of Neurology, Neurosurgery, and Psychiatry* 76 (2005): 103–105.

Jagust, W., D. Harvey, D. Mungas, and M. Haan. "Central Obesity and the Aging Brain." *Archives of Neurology* 62 (2005): 1545–1548.

Jonker, C., B. Schmand, J. Lindeboom, L. M. Havekes, and L. J. Launer. "Association Between Apolipoprotein E ε4 and the Rate of Cognitive Decline in Community-Dwelling Elderly Individuals With and Without Dementia." *Archives of Neurology* 55 (1998): 1065–1069.

Kalmijn, S., D. Foley, L. White, C. M. Burchfiel, J. D. Curb, H. Petrovitch, G. W. Ross, R. J. Havlik, and L. J. Launer. "Metabolic Cardiovascular Syndrome and Risk of Dementia in Japanese-American Elderly Men." *Arteriosclerosis, Thrombosis, and Vascular Biology* 20 (2000): 2255–2260.

Khachaturian, A. S., P. P. Zandt, C. G. Lyketsos, K. M. Hayden, I. Skoog, M. C. Norton, J. T. Tschanz, L. S. Mayer, K. A. Welsh-Bohmer, and J.C.S. Breitner. "Antihypertensive Medication Use and Incident Alzheimer Disease." *Archives of Neurology* 63 (2006): 686–692.

Korf, E.S.C., L. R. White, P. Scheltens, and L. J. Launer. "Midlife Blood Pressure and the Risk of Hippocampal Atrophy—The Honolulu Asia Aging Study." *Hypertension* 44 (2004): 29–34.

Kryscio, R. J., F. A. Schmitt, J. C. Salazar, M. S. Mendiondo, and W. R. Markesbery. "Risk Factors for Transitions from Normal to Mild Cognitive Impairment and Dementia." *Neurology* 66 (2006): 828–832.

Leslie, M. "This Is Your Brain . . . And This Is Your Brain on Calcium." *Science of Aging Knowledge Environment* 15 (2002): nS4.

Lindauer, R.J.L., M. Olff, E.P.M. van Meijel, I.V.E. Carlier, and B.P.R. Gersons. "Cortisol, Learning, Memory and Attention in Relation to Smaller Hippocampal Volume in Police Officers with Posttraumatic Stress Disorder." *Biological Psychiatry* 59 (2006): 171–177.

Lindstrom, H. A., T. Fritsch, G. Petot, K. A. Smyth, C. H. Chen, S. M. Debanne, A. J. Lerner, and R. P. Friedland. "The Relationships Between Television Viewing in Midlife and the Development of Alzheimer's Disease in a Case-Control Study." *Brain and Cognition* 58 (2005): 157–165.

Meerlo, P., M. Koehl, K. van der Borght, and F. W. Turek. "Sleep Restriction Alters the Hypothalamic-Pituitary-Adrenal Response to Stress." *Journal of Neuroendocrinology* 14 (2002): 397–402.

Moceri, V. M., W. A. Kukull, I. Emanuel, G. van Belle, and E. B. Larson. "Early-Life Risk Factors and the Development of Alzheimer's Disease." *Neurology* 54 (2000): 415–420.

Mok, V.C.T., A. Wong, W.W.M. Lam, Y. H. Fan, W. K. Tang, T. Kwok, A.C.F. Hui, and K. S. Wong. "Cognitive Impairment and Functional Outcome After Stroke Associated with Small Vessel Disease." *Journal of Neurology, Neurosurgery, and Psychiatry* 75 (2004): 560–566.

Mori, E., N. Hirono, H. Yamashita, T. Imamura, Y. Ikejiri, H. Ikeda, H. Kitagaki, I. Shimomura, and Y. Yoneda. "Premorbid Brain Size as a Determinant of Reserve Capacity Against Intellectual Decline in Alzheimer's Disease." *American Journal of Psychiatry* 154 (1997): 18–24.

Neumeister, A., D. S. Charney, and W. C. Drevets. "Depression and the Hippocampus." *American Journal of Psychiatry* 162 (2005): 1057.

Neumeister, A., S. Wood, O. Bonne, A. C. Nugent, D. A. Luckenbaugh, T. Young, E. E. Bain, D. S. Charney, and W. C. Drevets. "Reduced Hippocampal Volume in Unmedicated, Remitted Patients with Major Depression Versus Control Subjects." *Biological Psychiatry* 57 (2005): 935–937.

Ohm, T. G., F. Glockner, R. Distl, S. Treiber-Held, V. Meske, and B. Schonheit. "Plasticity and the Spread of Alzheimer's Disease-like Changes." *Neurochemistry Research* 28 (2003): 1715–1723.

Ong, W. Y., and A. A. Farooqui. "Iron, Neuroinflammation and Alzheimer's Disease." *Journal of Alzheimer's Disease* 8 (2005): 183–200.

Patel, N. V., M. N. Gordon, K. E. Connor, R. A. Good, R. W. Engelman, J. Mason, D. G. Morgan, T. E. Morgan, and C. E. Finch. "Caloric Restriction Attenuates Abeta-Deposition in Alzheimer Transgenic Animals." *Neurobiology of Aging* 26 (2005): 995–1000.

Persson, J., J. Lind, A. Larson, M. Ingvar, M. Cruts, C. Van Broeckhoven, R. Adolfsson, L. G. Nilsson, and L. Nyberg. "Altered Brain White Matter Integrity in Healthy Carriers of the APO E ε4 allele. A Risk for AD?" *Neurology* 66 (2006): 1029–1033.

Pruessner, J. C., M. W. Baldwin, K. Dedovic, R. Renwick, N. K. Mahani, C. Lord, M. Meaney, and S. Lupien. "Self-Esteem, Locus of Control, Hippocampal Volume and Cortisol Regulation in Young and Old Adulthood." *NeuroImage* 28 (2005): 815–826.

Ravaglia, G., P. Forti, F. Maioli, M. Martelli, L. Servadei, N. Brunetti, E. Porcellini, and F. Licastro. "Homocysteine and Folate as Risk Factors for Dementia and Alzheimer Disease." *American Journal of Clinical Nutrition* 82 (2005): 636–643.

Reynolds, E. H. "Folic Acid, Ageing, Depression and Dementia." *British Medical Journal* 324 (2002): 1512–1515.

Richards, M., and A. Sacker. "Lifetime Antecedents of Cognitive Reserve." *Journal of Clinical and Experimental Neuropsychology* 25 (2003): 614–624.

Rosenberg, P. B. "Clinical Aspects of Inflammation in Alzheimer's Disease." *International Review of Psychiatry* 17 (2006): 503–514.

Scarmeas, N., and Y. Stern. "Cognitive Reserve and Lifestyle." *Journal of Clinical and Experimental Neuropsychology* 25 (2003): 625–633.

Scheid, R., K. Walther, T. Guthke, C. Pruel, and Y. von Cramon. "Cognitive Sequelae of Diffuse Axonal Injury." *Archives of Neurology* 63 (2006): 418–424.

Schmidt, R., H. Schmidt, J. D. Curb, K. Masaki, L. R. White, and L. J. Launer. "Early Inflammation and Dementia: A 25 Year Follow-up of the Honolulu-Asia Aging Study." *Annals of Neurology* 52 (2002): 168–174.

Schupf, N., D. Kapell, J. H. Lee, R. Ottman, and R. Mayeux. "Increased Risk of Alzheimer's Disease in Mothers of Adults with Alzheimer's Disease." *Lancet* 344 (1994): 353–356.

Seshadri, S., A. Beiser, J. Selhub, P. F. Jacques, I. H. Rosenberg, R. B. D'Agostino, P.W.F. Wilson, and P. A. Wolf. "Plasma Homocysteine as a Risk Factor for Dementia and Alzheimer's Disease." *New England Journal of Medicine* 346 (2002): 476–483.

Volkow, N. D., J. Logan, J. S. Fowler, G. J. Wang, R. C. Gur, C. Wong, C. Felder, S. J. Gatley, Y. S. Ding, R. Hitzemann, and N. Pappas. "Association Between Age-Related Decline in Brain Dopamine Activity and Impairment in Frontal and Cingulate Metabolism." *American Journal of Psychiatry* 157 (2000): 75–80.

Watson, G. S., B. A. Cholerton, M. A. Reger, L. D. Baker, S. R. Plymate, S. Asthana, M. A. Fishel, J. J. Kulstad, P. S. Green, D. G. Cook, S. E. Kahn, M. L. Keeling, and S. Craft. "Preserved Cognition in Patients with Early Alzheimer Disease and Amnestic Mild Cognitive Impairment During Treatment with Rosiglitazone: A Preliminary Study." *American Journal of Geriatric Psychiatry* 13 (2005): 950–958.

Welberg, L.A.M., and J. R. Seckl. "Prenatal Stress, Glucocorticoids and the Programming of the Brain." *Journal of Neuroendocrinology* 13 (2001): 113–128.

Whitman, G. T., T. Tang, A. Lin, and R. W. Baloh. "A Prospective Study of Cerebral White Matter Abnormalities in Older People with Gait Dysfunction." *Neurology* 57 (2001): 990–994.

Zecca, L., M.B.H. Youdim, P. Riederer, J. R. Connor, and R. R. Crichton. "Iron, Brain Ageing and Neurodegenerative Disorders." *National Review of Neuroscience* 5 (2004): 863–873.

INDEX